PHOTO

An aid for the study of Physical Diagnosis

$$\boxed{1}$$

G S J Chessell, Dip Ed Tech.
*Coordinator, Medical Learning Resources Group,
University of Aberdeen*

M J Jamieson, MRCP
*Lecturer, Department of Therapeutics and Clinical
Pharmacology, University of Aberdeen*

R A Morton, MSc
*Director, Department of Medical Illustration,
University of Aberdeen*

J C Petrie, FRCP
*Reader, Department of Therapeutics and Clinical
Pharmacology, University of Aberdeen; Honorary
Consultant Physician, Aberdeen Teaching
Hospitals.*

H M A Towler, MRCP
*Lecturer, Department of Medicine,
University of Aberdeen.*

Year Book Medical Publishers, Inc.
Chicago

Photo Dix—an aid for the study of clinical diagnosis.

  Bibliography: P.
  Includes index.
  1. Diagnosis—Atlases. I. Chessell, G. S. J. (DNLM:
1. Diagnosis—Examination Questions. 2. Diagnosis,
Differential—Examination Questions. WB 18 P575)

RC71.3.P46 1984   616.07'5'076 84-17350
ISBN 0-8151-1653-5

Printed by Blantyre Printing and Binding Co Ltd

PHOTO D$_X$ — PREFACE

This is volume one of a four-volume series. PHOTO D$_X$ was designed as a study aid to test and improve your diagnostic skills over a wide range of clinical problems.

PHOTO D$_X$ features clinical photographs accompanied by questions that medical students and practising physicians should ask themselves during a patient interview to reach a diagnosis, or may be asked on medical school and board examinations. Answers are provided in a separate section of each volume.

As a part of the continuing education feature of this series, these questions and answers are designed to stimulate additional reading by both medical students and practitioners to further improve diagnostic skills.

The pictures in this new series have been selected from the clinical slide library in the Department of Medical Illustration, University of Aberdeen. The books have been produced against a background of experience gained over the last 10 years in the compilation for local use of over 2,000 self-assessment examples. The local exercise was coordinated through the Medical Learning Resources Group of the Faculty of Medicine, University of Aberdeen, in collaboration with many of the clinicians in the Aberdeen Teaching Hospitals.

The PHOTO D$_X$ series will be of interest to all who are committed to perfecting their skills in clinical diagnosis and to their own continuing medical education. We welcome comment on individual questions and answers.

Although numbering is sequential, each volume in the series is unique, containing a balanced selection of diagnostic examples, and thus may be used independently.

ACKNOWLEDGEMENTS

We wish to acknowledge the invaluable contribution of Dr Anthony Hedley, now Professor of Community Medicine, University of Glasgow, who was the instigator of the self-assessment program on which these books are based. We would also like to acknowledge the cooperation of all patients, secretarial and technical staff, in particular the staff of the Department of Medical Illustration, who have contributed in one way or another to the preparation of these volumes, and Mrs Margaret Doverty who typed the manuscript.

We would particularly like to thank the following colleagues for contributing material for the books:

Dr D R Abramovich, Mr A Adam, Mr A K Ah-See, Dr D J G Bain, Dr L S Bain, Dr K Bartlett, Dr A P Bayliss, Dr B Bennett, Miss F M Bennett, Dr P Best, Dr P D Bewsher, Mr C Birchall, Mr C T Blaiklock, Dr L J Borthwick, Mr P L Brunnen, Dr P W Brunt, Dr J Calder, Professor A G M Campbell, Dr B Carrie, Dr P Carter, Dr G R D Catto, Mr R B Chesney, Dr N Clark, Mr P B Clarke, Mr A I Davidson, Dr R J L Davidson, Dr A A Dawson, Mr W B M Donaldson, Professor A S Douglas, Dr A W Downie, Dr C J Eastmond, Mr J Engeset, Dr N Edward, Dr J K Finlayson, Dr J R S Finnie, Mr A V Foote, Dr N G Fraser, Mr R J A Fraser, Dr J A R Friend, Dr D B Galloway, Mr J M C Gibson, Dr D Hadley, Dr J E C Hern, Dr A W Hutcheon, Dr T A Jeffers, Dr A W Johnston, Mr P F Jones, Dr A C F Kenmure, Mr I R Kernohan, Dr A S M Khir, Mr J Kyle, Dr J S Legge, Mr McFadzean, Dr E McKay, Mr J McLauchlan, Mr K A McLay, Professor M MacLeod, Dr R A Main, Mr Mather, Mr N A Matheson, Mr J D B Miller, Mr S S Miller, Mr K L G Mills, Dr N A G Mowat, Mr I F K Muir, Dr L E Murchison, Mr W J Newlands, Mr J G Page, Professor R Postlethwaite, Dr J M Rawles, Mr P K Ray, Mr C R W Rayner, Professor A M Rennie, Mr A G R Rennie, Dr J A N Rennie, Dr O J Robb, Dr H S Ross, Dr G Russell, Dr D S Short, Dr P J Smail, Dr C C Smith, Professor G Smith, Dr L Stankler, Mr J H Steyn, Professor J M Stowers, Dr G H Swapp, Mr J Wallace, Professor W Walker, Dr S J Watt, Dr J Weir, Dr J Webster, Dr M I White, Dr F W Wigzell, Dr M J Williams, Mr L C Wills, Dr L A Wilson, Mr H A Young.

This thirty-five year old woman complained of tinnitus in her left ear. Clinical examination revealed an absent gag reflex and weakness of the soft palate, sternomastoid and trapezius on the left.
a What abnormality is seen in the middle ear?
b What is the most likely diagnosis?
c How should this condition be treated?

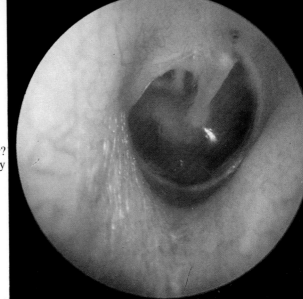

1

2 This is the bone-marrow aspirate smear of a thirty year old woman. Three months after returning from a holiday which involved travelling overland from Nepal to Turkey, she has developed biphasic diurnal fever, anaemia, splenomegaly, and recurrent epistaxis.
a What abnormality is present and which diagnosis does it indicate?
b Which vector is responsible for transmission of this disease?
c What drug therapy is appropriate?

2

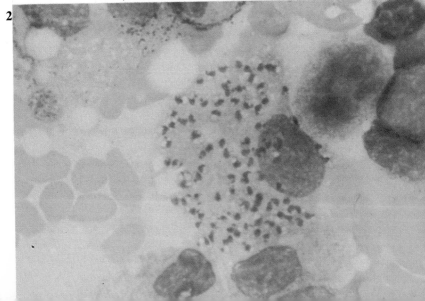

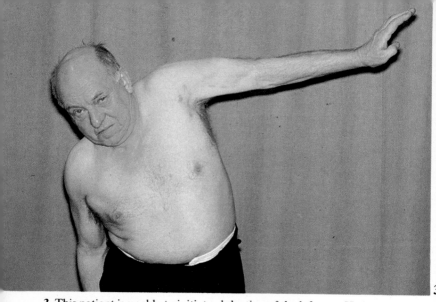

3 This patient is unable to initiate abduction of the left arm. He is, however, able to maintain abduction of the passively abducted arm, as seen here. What is the diagnosis?

4 a What is the likely cause of this patient's painful knee?
  b What common name is given to this condition?
  c Is the knee joint likely to be involved?

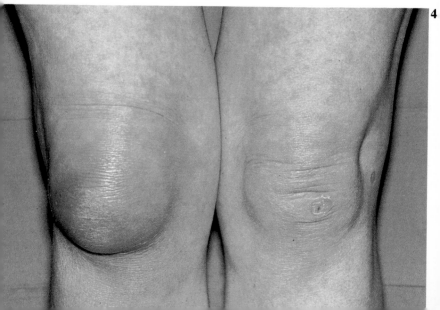

This seventy year old
patient gives a two month
history of temporal
headaches. He has been
aware of tenderness of the
scalp, especially when
combing his hair.
a What diagnosis does the
history suggest?
b Which symptoms and
which sign are regarded
as pathognomonic of this
disorder?
c What abnormalities are
seen in the picture?

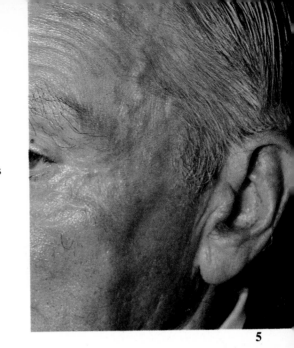

5

6

This patient is bedridden
because of severe
disseminated sclerosis. He
has recently developed mild
dependent oedema
associated with heavy
proteinuria (more than
three grammes/day) and
hypoalbuminaemia.
a What is the likely cause of
the lesions seen around
his right buttock?
b How might this explain
his proteinuria?
c What investigation would
you choose to establish
the diagnosis?

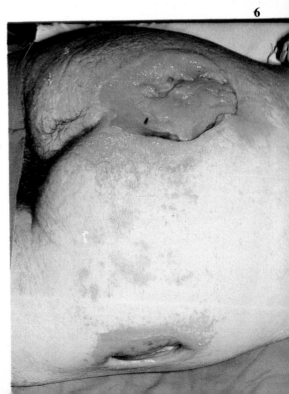

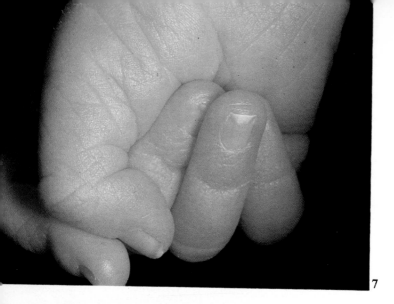

7

7 and 8 These abnormalities are characteristic of a chromosomal disorder.
a What name is given to the foot abnormality?
b What is the chromosomal disorder?
c What is the prognosis of this disorder?

8

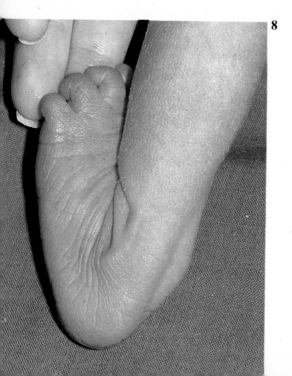

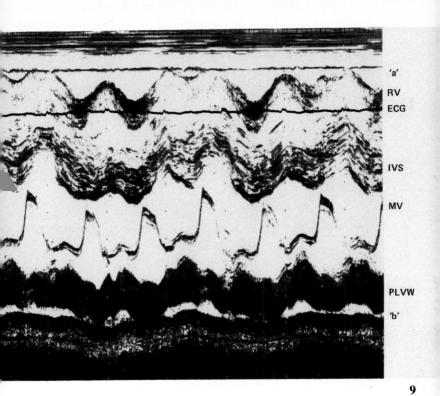

'a'
RV
ECG
IVS
MV
PLVW
'b'

9

9   RV   — right ventricular wall
      ECG   — electrocardiogram
      IVS   — interventricular septum
      MV   — mitral valve
      PLVW — posterior left ventricular wall

This M-mode echocardiogram is from a fourteen year old boy with
Hodgkin's disease.

a What is the cause of the echo-free spaces 'a' and 'b'?
b Which two other abnormalities are seen and what do these indicate?
c What urgent treatment may be necessary?

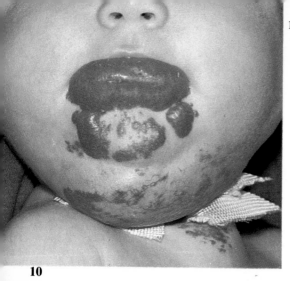

10 This lesion was not present at birth, but has gradually increased in size since then.
a What is the lesion?
b Give four reasons why specific treatment for such a lesion might be considered.

10

11

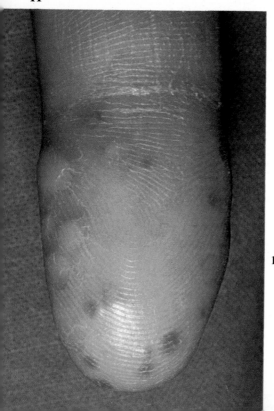

11 This nurse complains of painful lesions of her index finger.
a What are these lesions?
b What investigation is most helpful in establishing the diagnosis?

12 This patient complains of discomfort in his neck and axillae after drinking alcohol. He has recently become aware of a change in the appearance of his skin.
   a What name is given to the abnormal skin appearance?
   b What is the most likely underlying disorder?
   c List three other diseases associated with a similar skin abnormality.

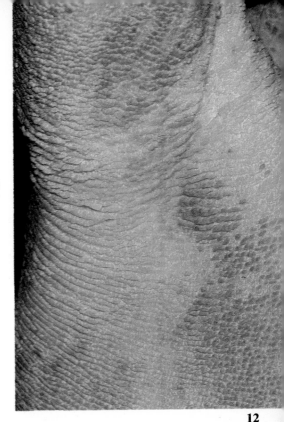

12

13 This patient's right pupil reacts to accommodation but not to light. The smaller left pupil reacts normally.
   a What name is given to the abnormal pupillary response?
   b This patient's pupillary reactions and appearances are typical of neurosyphilis — true or false?

13

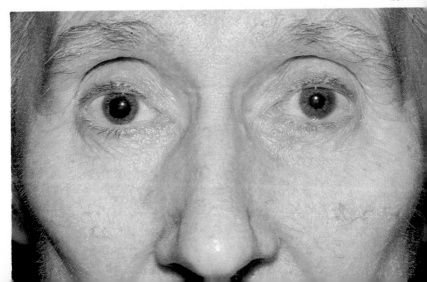

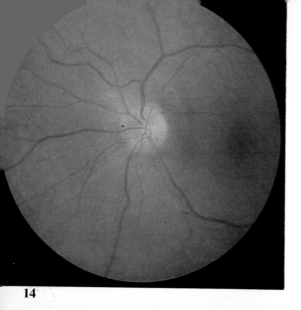

14 This patient complains of blurred vision. In order to focus on the retinal vessels, a normally-sighted examiner has to use a +10 dioptre lens.
  a What visual abnormality does this indicate?
  b What fundal abnormality is seen?

14

15

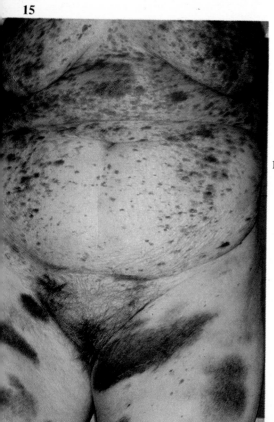

15 This seventy-six year old woman was treated with co-trimoxazole for a urinary tract infection. She complained of a sore throat a week before this appearance developed.
  a What is the probable diagnosis?
  b What clinical evidence would support this?
  c What would bone marrow aspiration show?
  d Which moiety of the co-trimoxazole is the likely culprit?

16, 17 and 18 This man presented with malaise, backache and deteriorating visual acuity. Haemoglobin was 8.8 g/dl and the erythrocyte sedimentation rate was 118mm. in the first hour.

a What radiological abnormalities are shown?

b What is the pathophysiology of the fundal appearance?

c What simple laboratory investigations are of great prognostic value?

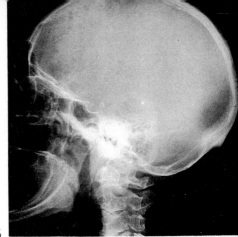

16

17

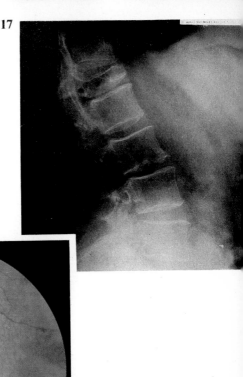

18

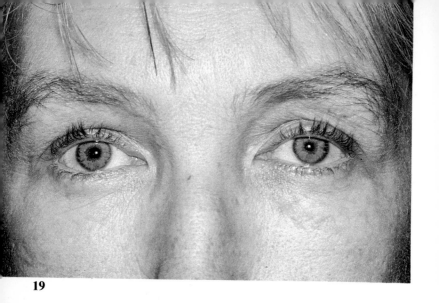

19

19 and 20 This patient's principal complaint is of pains across the shoulder girdle.
- a What abnormalities are seen in
  - i)   her face?
  - ii)   her hands?
- b Suggest two possible diagnoses.

20

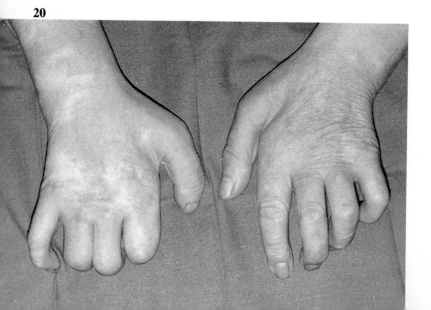

1 This patient has Graves' disease.
  a Which ocular feature is demonstrated here?
  b How is this abnormality measured objectively?

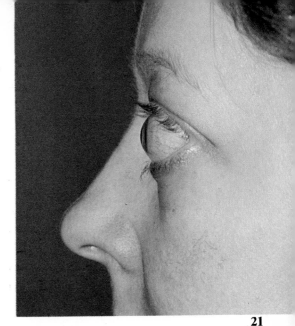

21

22

22 This patient has secondary amenorrhoea.
  a What changes are seen in her right breast?
  b What is the diagnosis?
  c When did she have her last period?

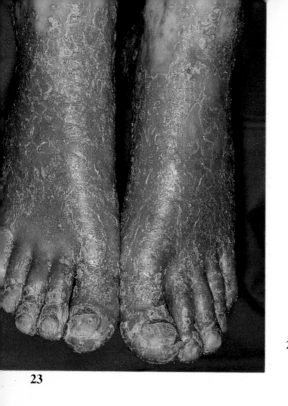

23

23 and 24 What metabolic
abnormality may these
patients have in common?

24

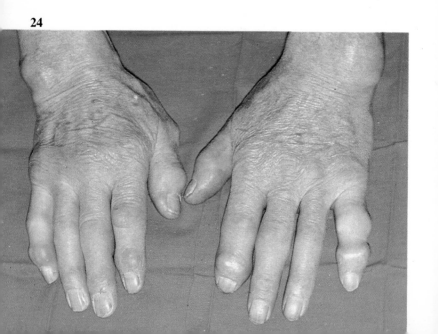

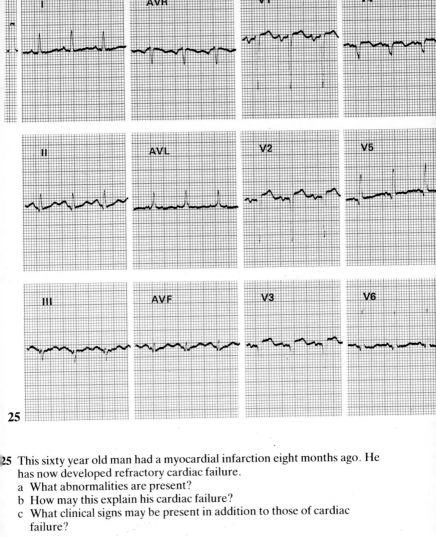

25

25 This sixty year old man had a myocardial infarction eight months ago. He has now developed refractory cardiac failure.
  a What abnormalities are present?
  b How may this explain his cardiac failure?
  c What clinical signs may be present in addition to those of cardiac failure?

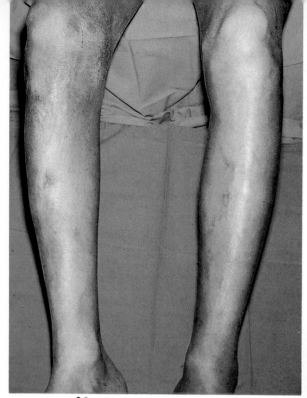

26

26 and 27 This patient complains of recurrent episodes of severe back pain, and, for years, of 'dragging' discomfort in his abdomen.

a What abnormalities are seen:
  i) on the skin of his legs?
  ii) in the x-ray of femur?
b What is the diagnosis?
c What is likely to be found on abdominal examination?
d Which biochemical abnormality is typical?

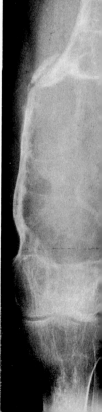

27

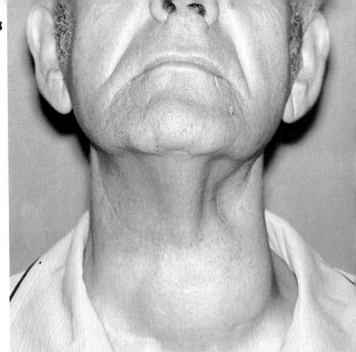

28 a Describe the principal abnormality shown.
 b Suggest three investigations which would help in making a diagnosis.
 c List three possible diagnoses.

29 This fifty-nine year old man with no previous history of bleeding
 problems presented with this appearance. The platelet count, bleeding
 time, thrombin time and prothrombin time were normal. The partial
 thromboplastin time was very long and not corrected by the addition of
 normal plasma or factor VIII.
 a What is the likely diagnosis?
 b In what conditions may this occur?

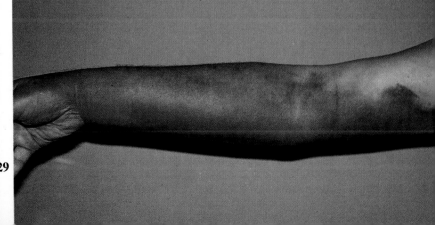

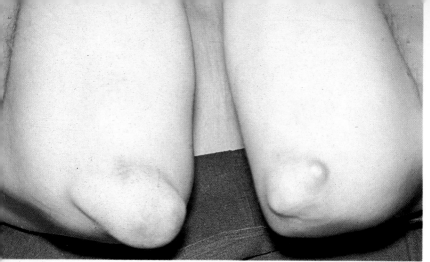

30

30 a What are these?
  b Where else do they occur?
  c What is their implication?

31

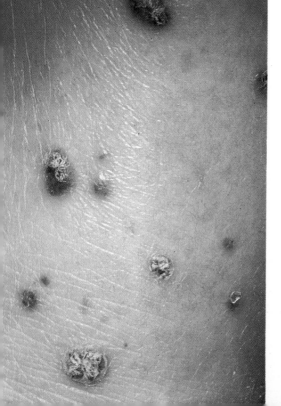

31 a What are these lesions?
  b What forms of treatment are available for such lesions?

32 This male patient was referred because of short stature.

   a What features are shown?
   b What is the likely diagnosis?
   c How can this be confirmed?

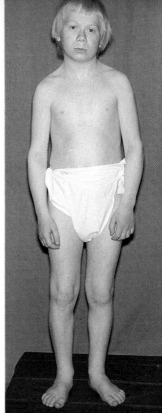

32

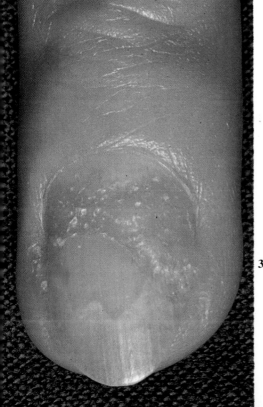

33 a What is the most likely diagnosis associated with the nail abnormalities shown?

   b What are the characteristic nail changes in this condition?

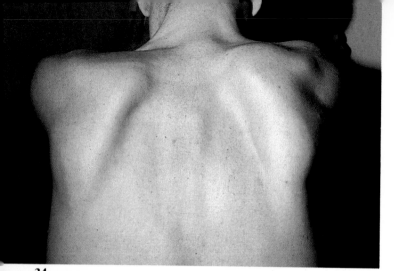

34

35

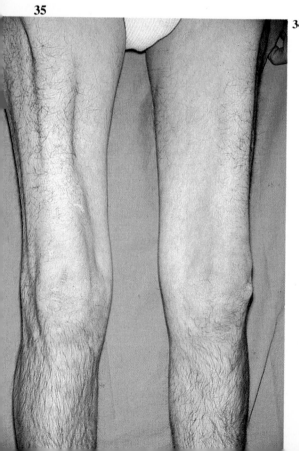

34 and 35 As a young man, this patient developed increasing weakness in his arms followed by proximal leg weakness. Limb-girdle dystrophy was diagnosed.

a Is he likely to be of low intelligence?

b Are the tendon reflexes normal in this condition?

c Is his life expectancy likely to be shortened?

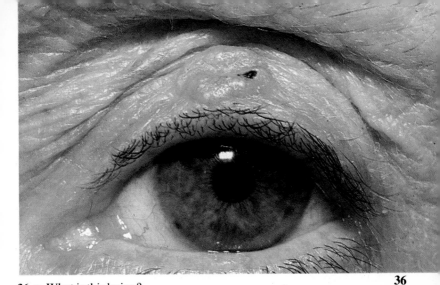

36 a What is this lesion?
   b What are the hazards of irradiating it?
   c What other therapies are available?

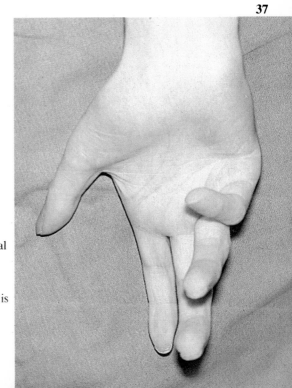

37 This man has a peripheral
   nerve lesion.
   a Which nerve is
     principally affected?
   b What unusual feature is
     present?
   c How can this be
     explained?

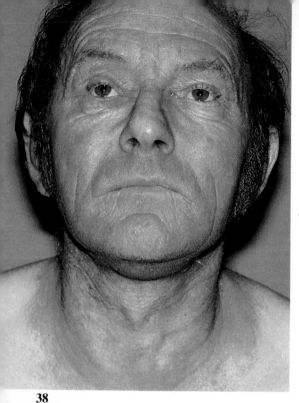

38 This patient is a maturity onset diabetic, and is hypertensive. His current regular medication includes amiloride, hydrochlorothiazide, nifedipine and chlorpropamide. Which of these drugs is/are most likely to be responsible for his skin rash?

39 This child suffers from chronic anaemia, recurrent infections and (until a recent surgical procedure) a severe bleeding tendency. During an acute respiratory illness the following results were obtained: Haemoglobin 3.5 g/dl. Blood film — hypochromia and considerable variation in red cell size, with red cell fragments; reticulocytosis accompanied by large numbers of nucleated red cells; polymorph

38

39

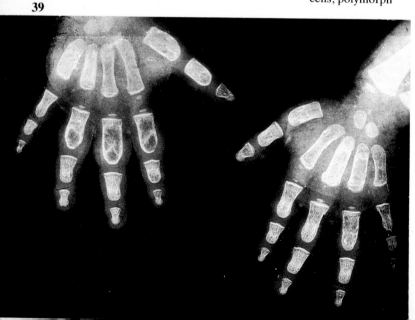

leucocytosis; platelet count normal.

a What abnormality is seen in the x-ray of the hands?

b What is the most likely diagnosis?

c Which surgical procedure was performed?

d Which complication of this procedure may have developed?

This lesion was present at birth and has slowly enlarged since.

a What is the likely diagnosis?

b What is the principal significance of such lesions?

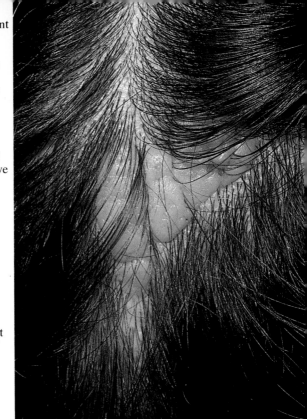

40

41 This patient's I.Q. is sixty.

a What ocular abnormality is seen?

b What is the diagnosis?

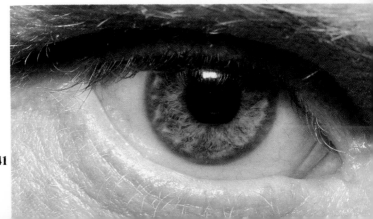

41

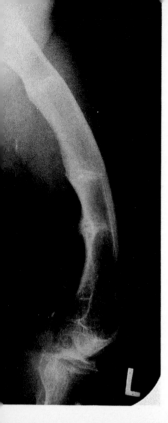

42 This patient is on regular
treatment for epilepsy.
  a What abnormalities are
    seen in the x-ray of his
    femur?
  b What is the cause?
  c How does this relate to
    his epilepsy?

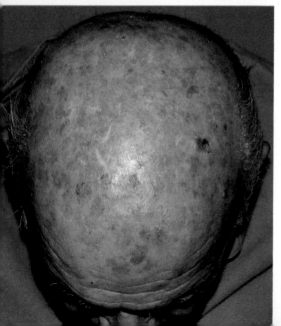

43 This patient has spent
several years in Australia.
  a What is the most likely
    cause of the scalp
    abnormality seen?
  b What is the significance
    of this condition?

43

44 What is the most likely cause of the asymptomatic lesions seen on this patient's thigh?

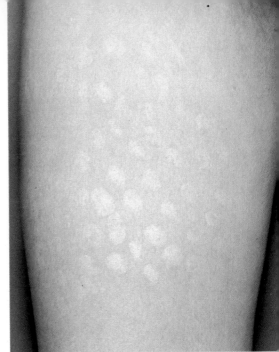

44

45

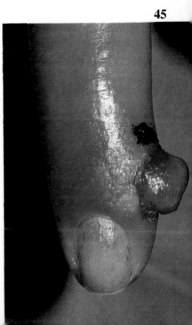

45 This lesion has increased in size rapidly over the past ten days. It has a tendency to bleed after minimal trauma.
   a What is the likely diagnosis?
   b What principal histological feature is typical?

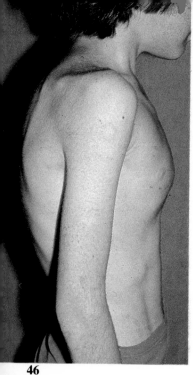

46 and 47

    a What abnormality of this child's chest is seen?

    b What is the most likely cause of his skin rash?

    c List three ocular disorders associated with the skin condition.

46

47

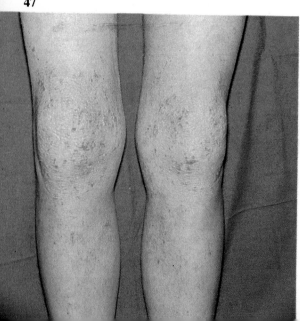

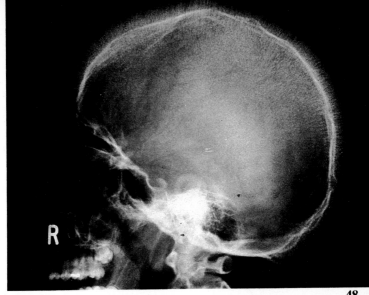

48 a What descriptive name is given to the radiological abnormality seen here?
 b What pathological process underlies the x-ray changes?
 c What is the most likely underlying condition?

49 This patient presented with redness and itching of the axillae. Sensitivity to deodorant was diagnosed and a topical cream was prescribed. Application of the cream produced initial relief, but once therapy was stopped the itching returned and the rash became more widespread. Despite continued treatment with the cream the rash has continued to spread.
 a What name is given to this condition?
 b What is its cause?

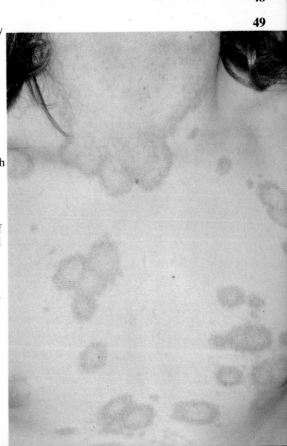

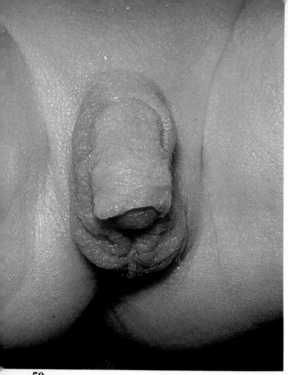

50

50 This baby's serum electrolytes include the following results. Sodium 120 mmol/l; potassium 5.6 mmol/l, bicarbonate 17 mmol/l; urea 9.0 mmol/l. Urinary sodium 40 mmol/l.

a What abnormality is demonstrated?

b Which diagnosis does the biochemistry and this appearance suggest?

c What is the likely biochemical defect?

51

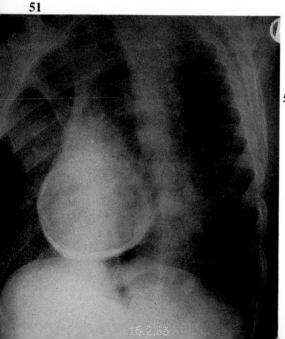

51 This patient presented with increasing tiredness and ankle oedema.

a What clinical abnormalities may be detected in the abdomen?

b What should be looked for on measuring her blood pressure?

c What may inspection of the jugular venous pulse reveal?

d What treatment is indicated?

52 and 53 This twenty-one year old male homosexual complained of a painful swollen left ankle. He had no urinary symptoms or recent alteration of bowel habit. Gram stain of joint aspirate showed intracellular Gram negative diplococci.

a What abnormalities are seen of his
  i) ankle?
  ii) feet?
b What is the most likely cause of his symptoms?
c How else should the diagnosis be established?

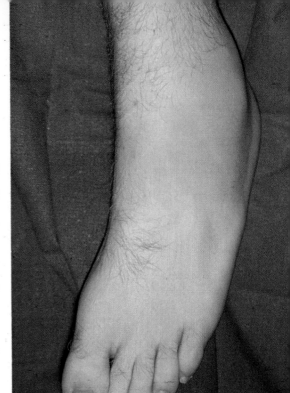

52

53

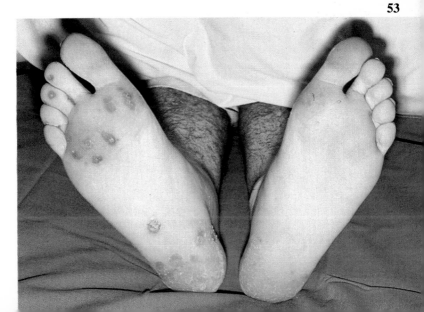

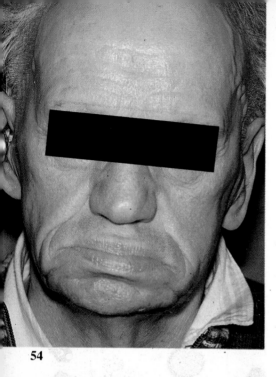

54 This patient has Huntington's chorea. His twenty-eight year old daughter is sixteen weeks pregnant.
  a What is the risk that her child will have the disorder?
  b How is the diagnosis established antenatally?
  c Which hepatic disorder is typically associated with this disease?

54

55

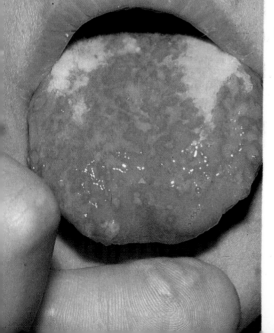

55 This child presented with fever, sore mouth and throat.
  a What abnormalities are shown on the anterior aspect of the tongue and thumb?
  b What is the likely diagnosis?
  c How could the oral and skin lesions be connected?

56 This patient suffers from chronic hepatocellular disease. Over the past two months he has lost three stones in weight and has complained of right upper quadrant pain. Abdominal examination reveals hepatomegaly, as delineated in pen, and an unusual auscultatory finding.
  a Suggest what the auscultatory finding may be.
  b What is your diagnosis?
  c List three factors which may predispose to this condition.

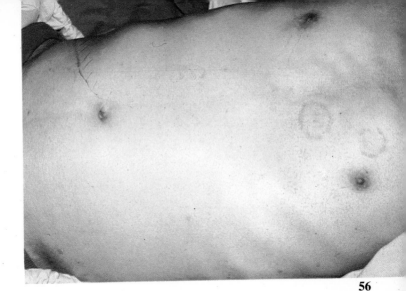

56

57

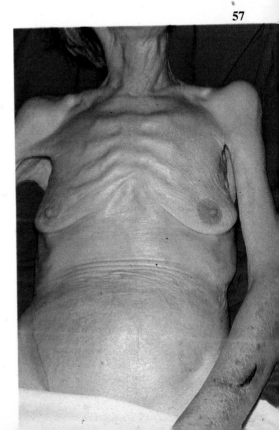

7 This patient was admitted following a haematemesis. Endoscopy revealed gastric erosions (probably related to recent ingestion of a nonsteroidal anti-inflammatory drug) but no other abnormality. She gave a history of four stones weight loss over the past two years but had no other abdominal symptoms. Haemoglobin was 8g/dl. The report on blood film was "hypochromic, microcytic anaemia. Howell Jolly bodies present". Barium meal showed no abnormality but flocculation of the barium column was observed on follow through.

a What is the most likely diagnosis?

b How does this explain the abnormal red cell features?

c What are the principal intestinal complications of this disorder?

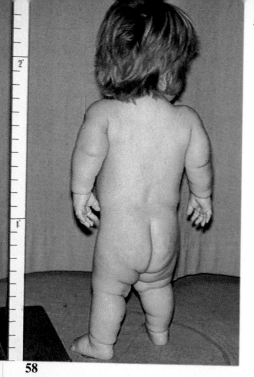

58 This child was born to normal parents.
  a What is this condition?
  b Which ossification process is abnormal?
  c What factor is associated with spontaneous cases of this disease?

58

59

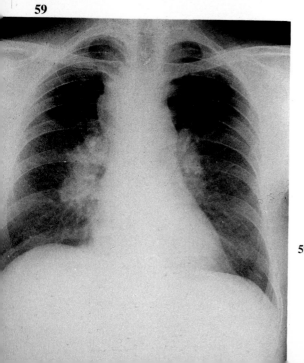

59 a What abnormality is shown?
  b What feature suggests that this is non-neoplastic?

60 and 61
a What is the most likely nature of the abnormalities seen in this patient's ear and ring finger?
b In which tissue are such lesions never found?
c Suggest three means by which this disorder may impair renal function.

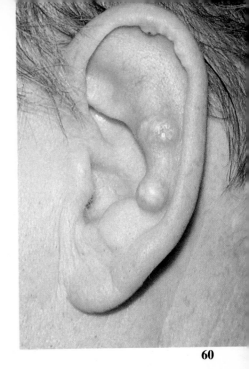

60

61

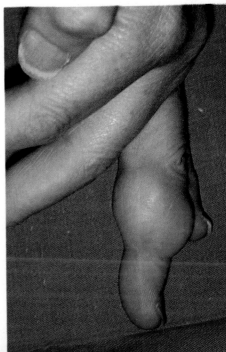

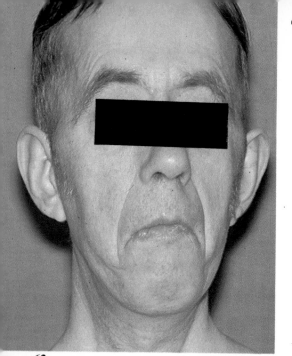

62 a What abnormal features
are shown here?
  b What is the likely
diagnosis?

62

63

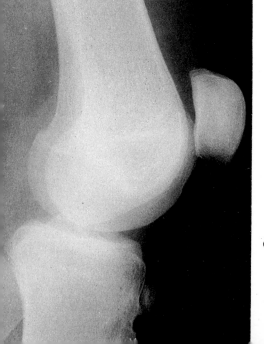

63 This young girl complains
of recurrent pain in and
swelling of the knee.
What is the diagnosis?

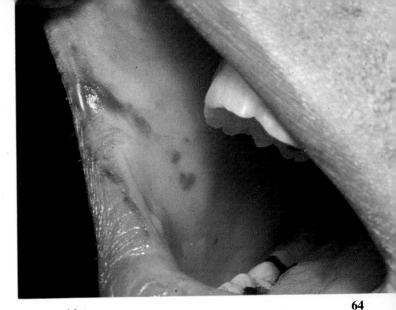

64

65

64 This patient presents with a history of weight loss, tiredness and blackouts.

a What two mucosal abnormalities are shown here?

b State the likely diagnosis.

c How can this be confirmed?

d List three important underlying causes of this disorder.

65 What should be suspected as the cause of this non-obese patient's iron deficiency anaemia?

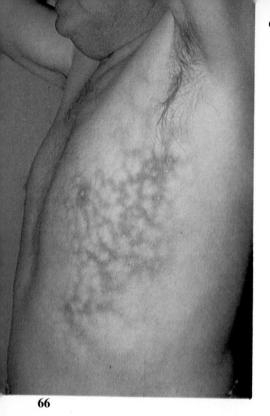

66 This patient complains of long-standing left sided chest pain.
a What name is given to the skin abnormality seen?
b What is its cause?

66

67 This thirty-eight year ol woman has angina pectoris.
a What abnormality is shown?
b What is its significan here?

67

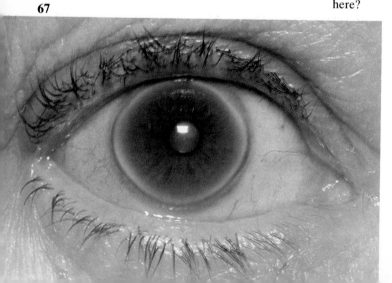

8 This patient became acutely dyspnoeic shortly after a diagnostic procedure was carried out on a general medical ward.
a What name is given to the appearance seen here?
b Which diagnostic procedure was performed?

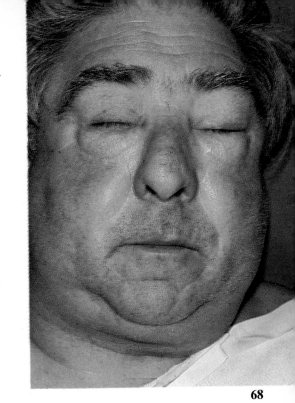

68

9 This patient, who has recently developed a symmetrical polyarthropathy affecting hands and feet, now complains of altered sensation over both feet, and of a 'drop foot' on the left. The lesions shown here were preceded by painless reddish black spots in the same sites.
a What are the lesions shown?
b What is the likely underlying joint disorder?
c What is the likely cause of her neurological symptoms?

69

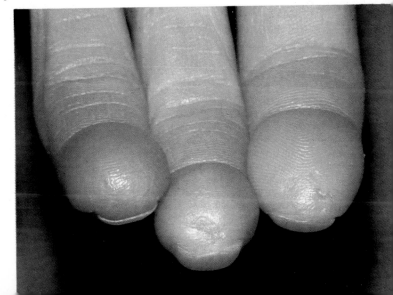

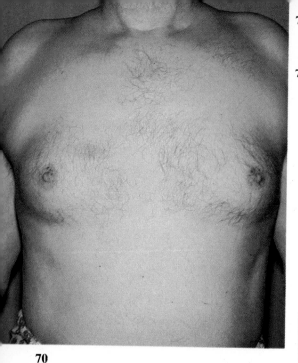

70

70 List six drugs which may give rise to this appearance in a male patient.

72 a What is the likely nature of the lesions seen under this patient's tongue?
b List four possible predisposing factors.

71 This fifty year old woman required replacement of a Bjork-Shiley aortic valve prosthesis when it jammed open because of a failure of anticoagulation.
a What signs would suggest this diagnosis?
b What complication of surgery has occurred?
c How was it treated?

71

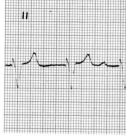

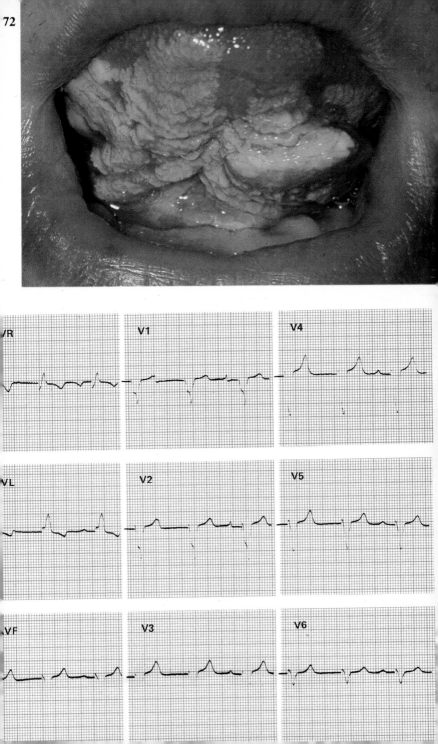

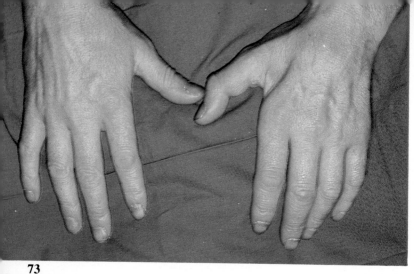

73

73 and 74 This patient has been referred for assessment of atypical angina pectoris.
  a What abnormality is seen in the hands?
  b What abnormalities are seen on chest x-ray?
  c What is the cause of his chest pain?

74

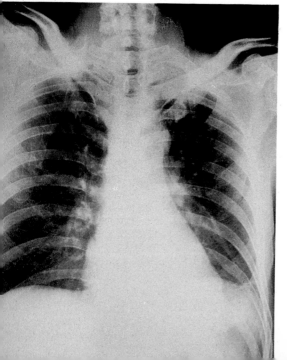

75 This seventy year old patient complains of altered sensation in the skin of his feet and legs. He has patchy sensory loss in both legs, weakness of foot eversion, ankle dorsiflexion on both sides, and of foot inversion on the left. His current medication includes hydralazine 25 mg twice daily. Urinalysis reveals traces of blood and protein but no other abnormality.

a What cutaneous abnormality is seen?

b What is the cause of the neurological symptoms and signs?

c What is the likely diagnosis in a patient of this age and sex?

d What blood test abnormalities would support this diagnosis?

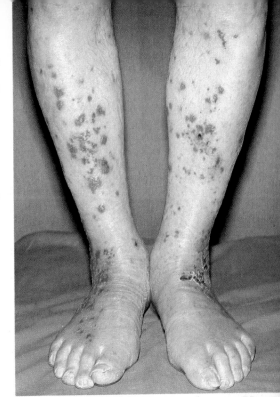

75

76

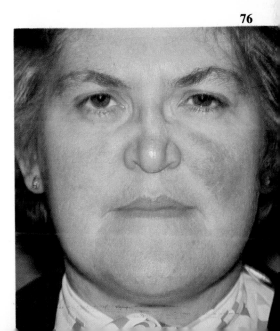

76 a What two abnormalities are visible on this patient's face?

b What are the two principal differential diagnoses?

c What simple bedside investigation may differentiate between the two?

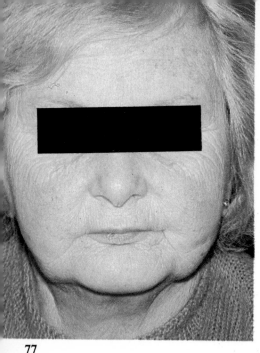

77 This patient is receiving thyroxine replacement therapy. She complains of cold intolerance.
  a Which physical sign best correlates with inadequate replacement?
  b Which single biochemical investigation is the most useful guide to adequacy of replacement in primary hypothyroidism?

77

78

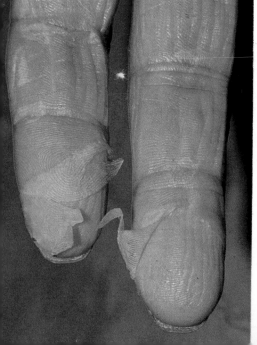

78 This abnormality developed two weeks after this patient had a sore throat.
  a Which infectious cause of sore throat is typically associated with this appearance?
  b What are the principal non-suppurative complications of this infection?

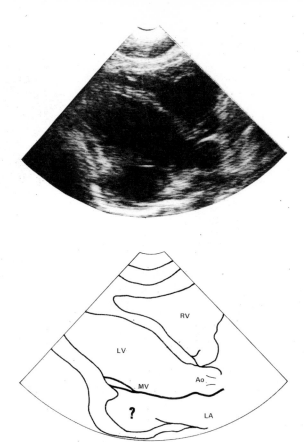

79

79 This cross-sectional echocardiogram is from a forty-five year old man who
has an abnormal ECG. Following an episode of prolonged retrosternal
and interscapular pain eight weeks ago, he has complained of exertional
dyspnoea and orthopnoea.
a What abnormality is seen on the echocardiogram (subcostal four-
chamber view)?
b What abnormalities may be present on his ECG?
c Which cardiac murmur may be present?

      RV   Right ventricle
      LV   Left ventricle
      MV Mitral valve
      Ao   Aorta
      LA   Left atrium

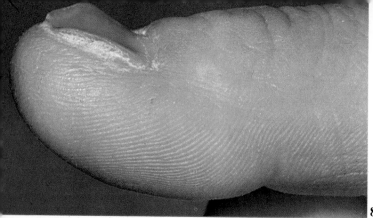

80 This patient complains of dysphagia.
  a What abnormality is shown?
  b How may this relate to the complaint?

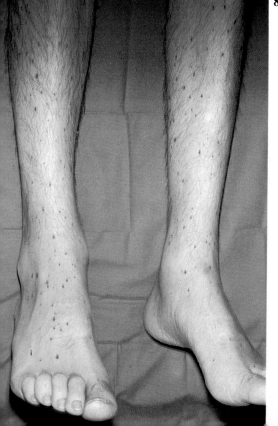

81 This patient's peripheral blood film is abnormal.
  a What abnormality should be sought on abdominal examination?
  b What diagnostic value would this abnormality have?
  c If abdominal examination is normal, what is the likely finding on histology of bone marrow aspirate?

82 a What is this condition?
b What are the
complications of this
condition?

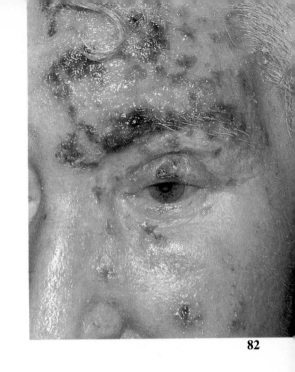

82

83

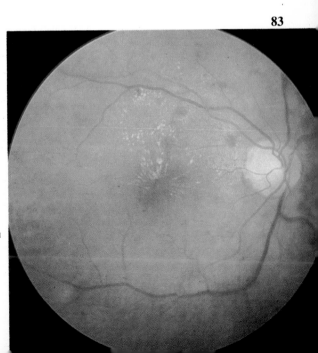

Describe the
abnormalities shown in
this optic fundus.
State the underlying
disorder.

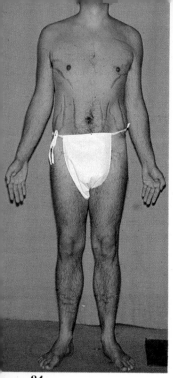

84

84 and 85 These patients are suffering from the same condition. They have undergone the same abdominal surgical operation.
  a What two abnormalities are seen in the male patient's skin?
  b What neurological abnormality does the female patient have?
  c What diagnosis is common to both?

85

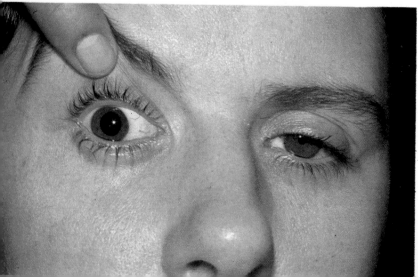

This man has chronic lymphocytic leukaemia.
a What is the origin of the abnormal cell line?
b What abnormalities of gamma globulins may be found in this disease?
c What are the two major causes of anaemia in this disease?
d What characteristic chromosomal abnormality is often present?

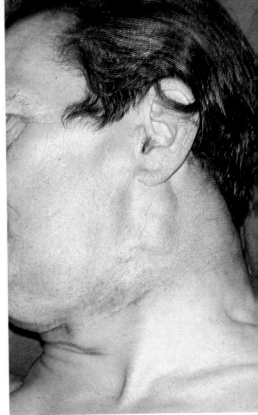

86

This patient has primary osteoarthrosis.
a What names are given to the swellings seen in
   i)   the distal interphalangeal joints?
   ii) the proximal interphalangeal joints?
b What is the nature of the swelling?

87

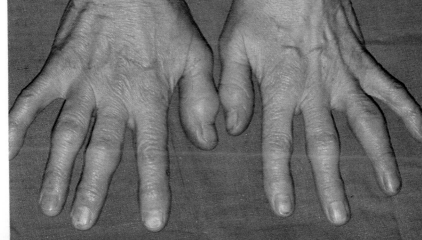

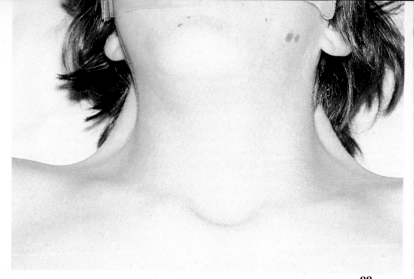

88

88 This patient has a congenital cardiovascular lesion.
   a What underlying problem is suggested by the appearance of her neck?
   b What clinical features of the cardiovascular lesion may be present?

89 Since a fall on outstretched hands three months ago this patient complains
   of persistent pain at the base of the thumb.
   What two abnormalities are seen in these x-rays?

89

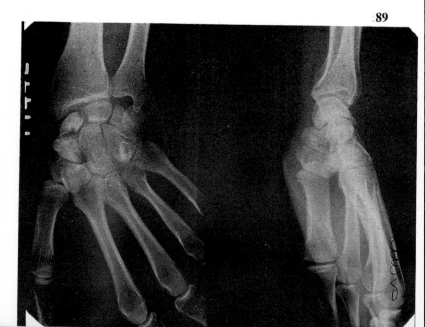

a Describe three
  abnormalities present.
b What is the diagnosis?

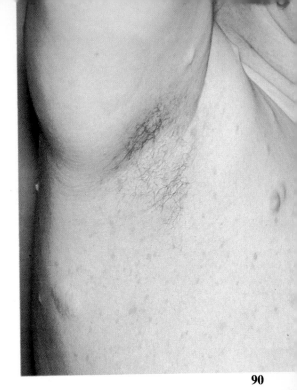

90

91 a What is the cause of this patient's itchy rash?
   b Which drug is most suitable for treatment of the rash?

91

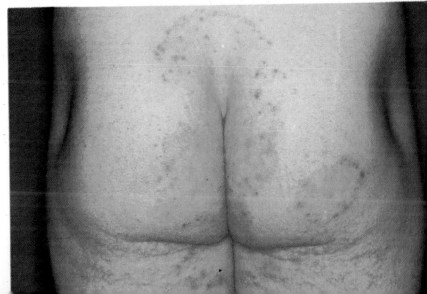

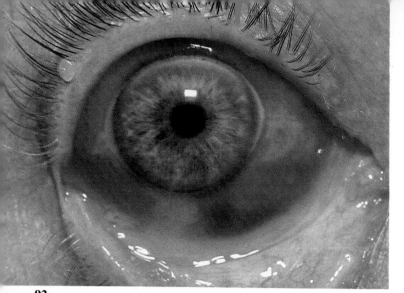

92

93

92 This thirty-nine year old man was knocked out in a road traffic accident. He was fully alert when seen initially but his conscious level deteriorated over the subsequent two hours. By the time of his arrival in hospital he had generalised increased muscle tone and bilateral extensor plantar responses.

a What diagnosis does his appearance suggest?

b What action is indicated?

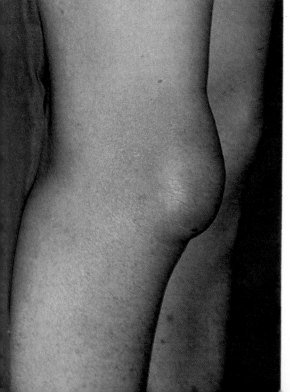

93 a What is this condition?

b Which organism is usually responsible?

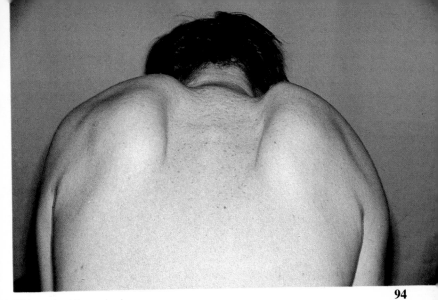

94

95

94 This patient has spinal muscular atrophy.
  a What features may help differentiate it from motor neurone disease?
  b What is the mainstay of treatment?

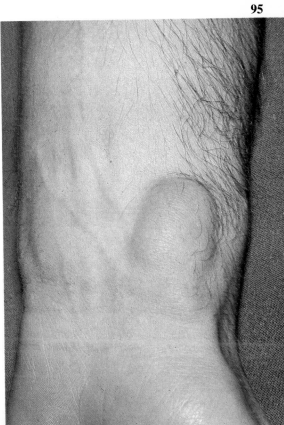

95 This man complains of a painless swelling on his wrist.
  a What is the likely diagnosis?
  b From what structure does it arise?
  c Is "text-book treatment" effective?

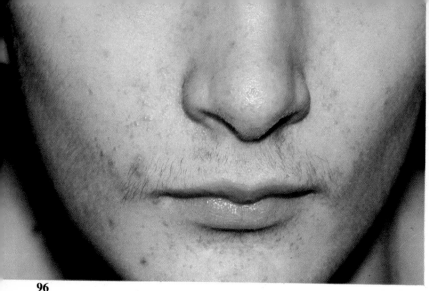

96

96 and 97 This patient has epilepsy. He is of average intelligence.
  a What underlying diagnosis is suggested by his facies? What name is given to the facial lesions?
  b What abnormalities are seen in the skin of his trunk?
  c What is the usual cause of epilepsy in this condition?
  d What two other skin abnormalities are typical of this disorder?

97

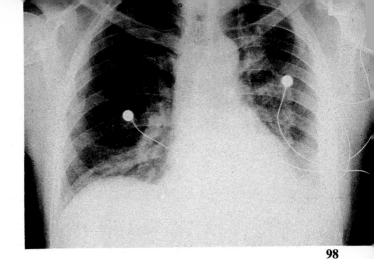

98

99

98 This x-ray was taken
during a routine medical
check up. The patient is
free of symptoms and has
no previous history of
acute respiratory or cardiac
illness.
  a What principal
     abnormality is seen on
     chest x-ray?
  b What is the most likely
     cause?
  c List three other
     respiratory
     complications of the
     underlying cause.

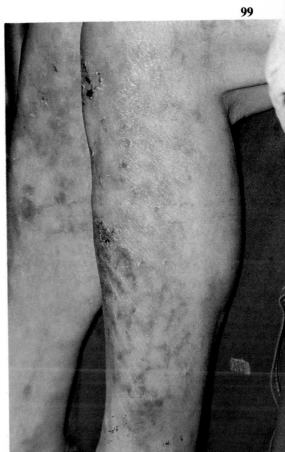

99 a What name is given to
       this rash?
   b What is the causative
       agent?
   c Does malignant
       transformation occur in
       these lesions?
   d What underlying
       medical disorder should
       be considered?

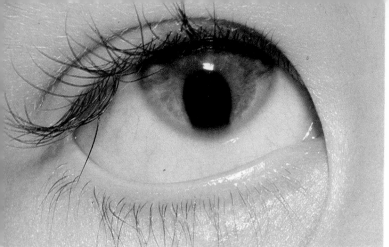

100

100 a What name is given to this abnormality?
b What is the cause?
c What is its significance

101

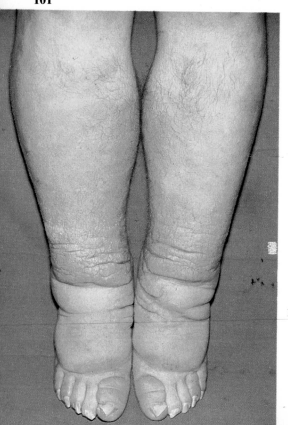

101 a What is this?
b What is the underlying diagnosis?
c What treatment is available for the condition shown?

102 Following a Mediterranean holiday this patient was disappointed by his rather patchy suntan. Since the suntan has faded he is aware of patchy areas of increased pigmentation.

a What is the name given to this condition?

b What is the cause?

c How may the diagnosis be established?

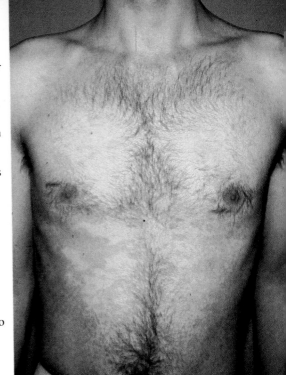

102

103 This lady was admitted to hospital in a toxic, confused state.

a What abnormality is shown here?

b What is the causative agent?

c What is its significance in relation to her presenting complaint?

103

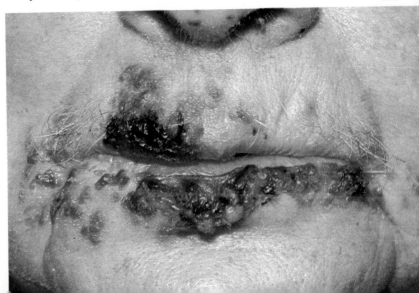

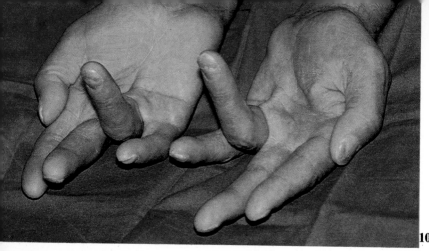

104 a A pattern of inheritance has been associated with this sign. What is it?

 b What neurological disorder has been associated with this sign?

105 and 106 The itching eruption seen over this patient's wrists developed over the course of two days.

 a How would you describe the skin lesions?

 b What is the most likely diagnosis?

 c What is the significance of buccal involvement in this condition?

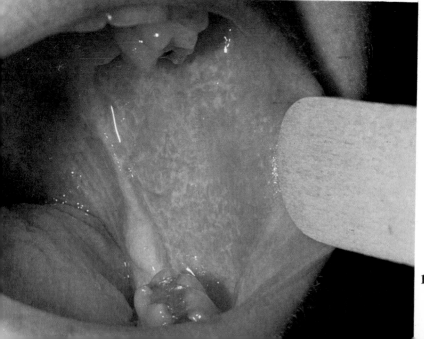

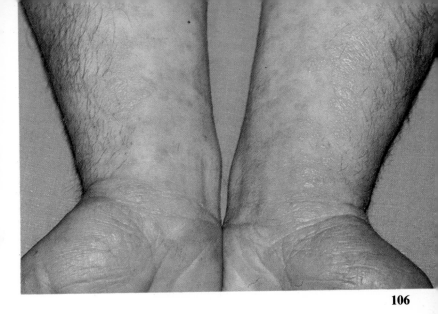

107 This patient sustained a right-sided stroke two months ago. Of what visual problem may he complain?

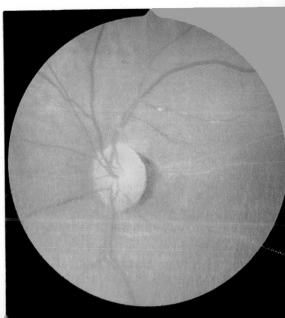

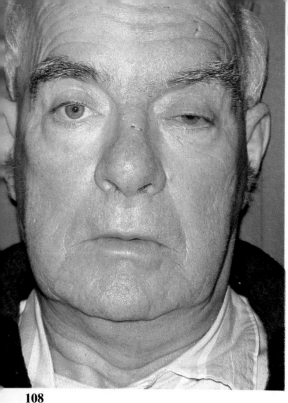

108 This man complained of pain above his left eye for several days before this appearance developed.
a What is the diagnosis?
b What is the significance of involvement of the nasociliary nerve in this disease?
c What therapies are useful?

108

109

109 This child's complaint of difficulty in rising from bed for some time was attributed to laziness.
a What abnormalities are seen in the chest x-ray?
b What is the most likely underlying diagnosis?

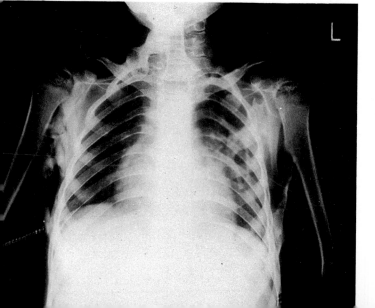

0 This patient complains of itchy spots around the ankle, which become swollen when rubbed. On a number of occasions she has experienced palpitations and lightheadedness shortly after scratching the ankle.

a What is the diagnosis?

b What histological abnormality is typical?

c What is the cause of her systemic symptoms?

d Which drugs should she avoid?

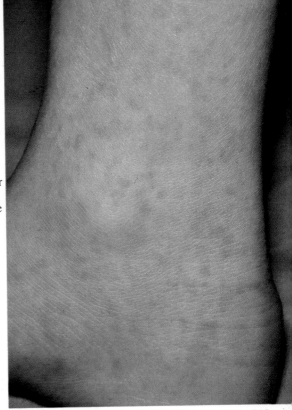

110

111 The lesion on this patient's forehead has increased rapidly in size over the past two to three weeks.

a What is the most likely diagnosis?

b What is the principal differential diagnosis?

111

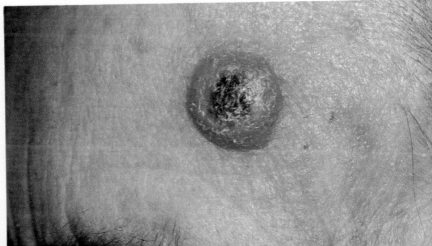

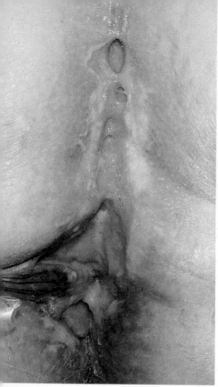

112

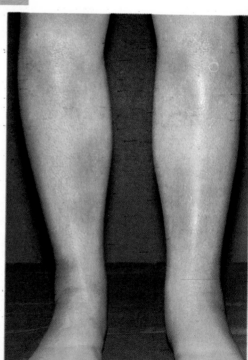

113

112 and 113 This patient has a ten year history of numerous surgical procedures to large and small bowel.

a What principal abnormality is shown?

b What is the underlying diagnosis?

c List four other alimentary causes for the skin lesions.

14 a What is likely to be this
    patient's principal
    complaint?
  b What drug treatment is
    most likely to be
    helpful?

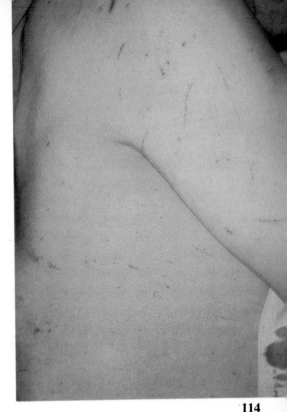

114

115

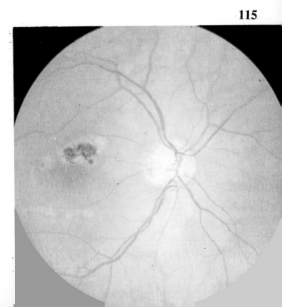

115 This seventy year old
    patient complains of
    gradually failing vision.
  a What principal
    abnormality is seen in
    the optic fundus?
  b What is the most likely
    cause of his visual
    deterioration?
  c Which structure is
    primarily affected?

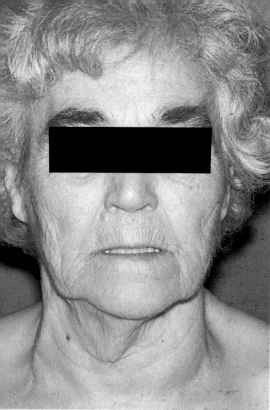

116 This patient with long standing anaemia give two month history of weight loss and epigas fullness after meals. She has a left-sided pt

a What abnormality i seen in her neck?

b How does this relat the eyelid abnorma

c How might these re to her presenting symptoms?

116

117 a What is this condition

b What are the clinical features of this disorder?

117

18 a What is the
   abnormality?
 b What does it indicate?

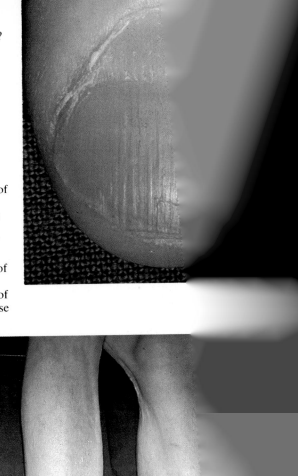

19 This patient complains of
   severe pain above the
   right knee joint and has
   recently lost weight.
   a What abnormality of
     the shins is shown?
   b What are the causes of
     this?
   c Which complication of
     the commoner of these
     may have occurred?

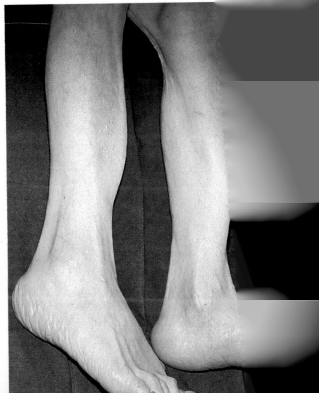

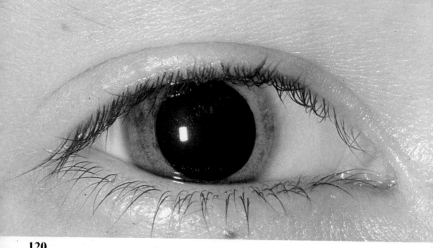

120 and 121 This child suffers from an unusual, inherited disorder
of mesenchymal tissue. He is tall for his age, with disproportionately
long extremities.
   a What name is given to the abnormal appearance of the hands?
   b What ocular abnormality is seen?
   c What is the diagnosis and how is it usually inherited?
   d Which disorder of metabolism may have similar clinical features?

121

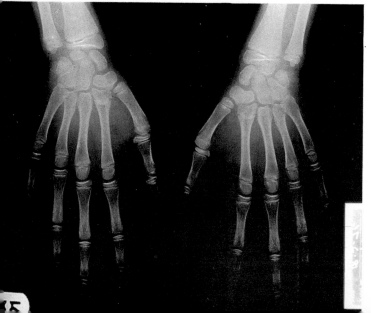

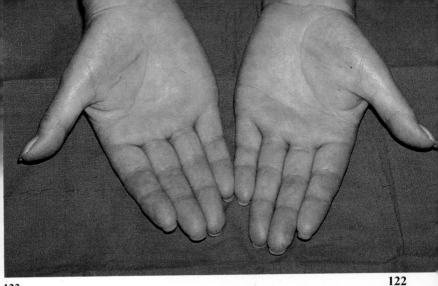

122

a What abnormality is
seen in the skin of these
hands?

b List five conditions
which may be
associated with these
appearances.

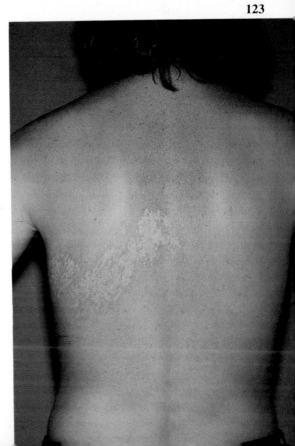

123

This young patient
complains of recurrent
lancinating pains under
his left shoulder and
anteriorly in his left lower
chest.

What is the most likely
cause?

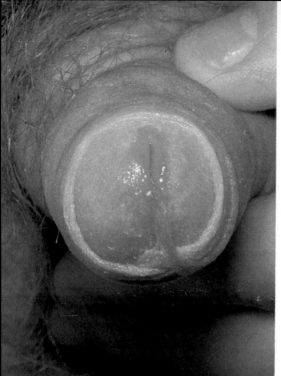

124

124 and 125 This patient complains of dysuria and of painful heels.

  a What abnormalities are seen on the x-ray?

  b What is the most likely diagnosis?

125

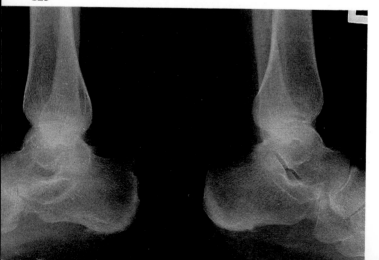

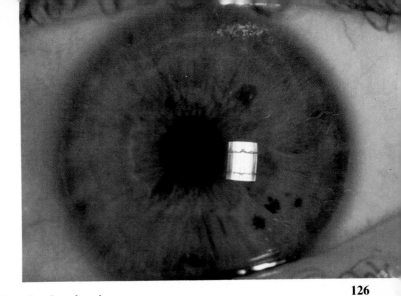

126 This patient has chronic
renal failure.
  a What is the
     abnormality?
  b What surgical
     procedure may be
     necessary?

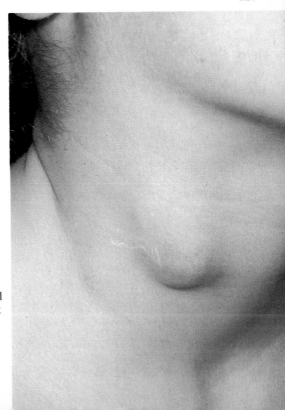

127 a Name two differential
        diagnoses of this neck
        swelling.
     b How is the diagnosis
        established?

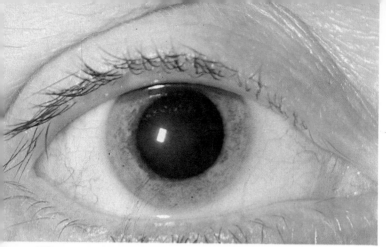

128

129

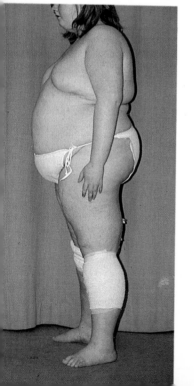

128 This forty-two year old
woman complains of
failing visual acuity.
a What ocular
abnormality is visible?
b What is the most likely
underlying cause?
c List four other ocular
features of this
disorder.

129 This obese seventeen year
old girl has Prader-Willi
syndrome.
a List four other features
of this disease.
b Name three other
conditions which may
have similar features.

130

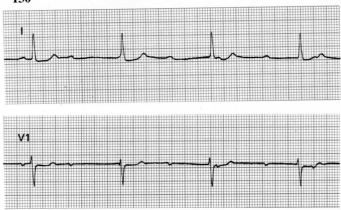

130 This asymptomatic thirty year old man was noted to have a bradycardia
at an insurance medical. An ECG was performed.
  a What rhythm is shown?
  b What is the probable aetiology?
  c Which further investigation would help establish the diagnosis?
  d What treatment is indicated?

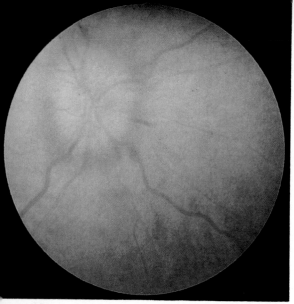

131 This is the fundus of a climber who complained of nausea, headache and unsteadiness after ascending 1,000m to 5,500m.
a What fundal abnormality is present?
b What is the diagnosis and which complication is developing?
c What treatment is indicated?

131

132

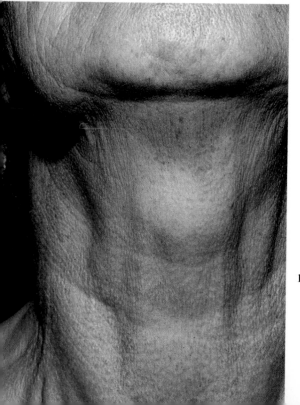

132 This swelling moves upward when the tongue is protruded.
a What is the diagnosis?
b From which pharyngeal pouch does it arise?

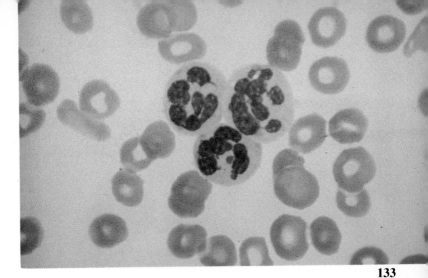

133

133 This is the blood film of a fifty year old woman who complained of poor balance, particularly in the dark, and tingling toes. Physical examination showed Rombergism, absent ankle and knee reflexes and extensor plantar responses.
  a What two abnormalities are present in the blood film?
  b Which diagnosis is suggested by the film appearance and clinical description?
  c List three other neurological complications of this condition.

134 This taxi-driver was assaulted by his passenger.
  a What three abnormalities are present?
  b What is the diagnosis?

134

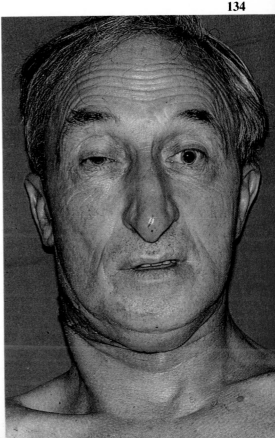

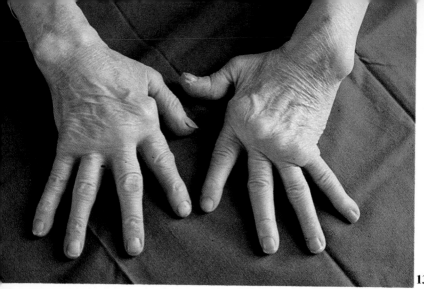

135

135 a List five abnormalities seen in these hands.
 b What is the likely diagnosis?
 c What principal complication is associated with the appearance of the distal ulna?

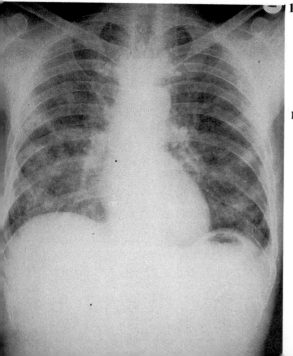

136

136 This pigeon breeder complains of cough and breathlessness of twelve months' duration. Bird fancier's lung is suspected.
 a Describe the radiological abnormalities.
 b Which investigations may help establish this diagnosis?
 c List eight industrial forms of extrinsic allergic alveolitis.

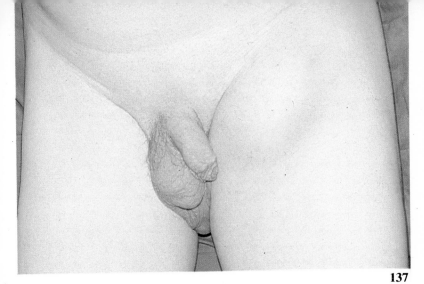

137

137 What is the differential diagnosis of the swelling in this six year old child's groin?

138 This sixty-four year old lady has chronic obstructive airways disease. Name the structures labelled 1 to 5 on the CT scan through the chest.

138

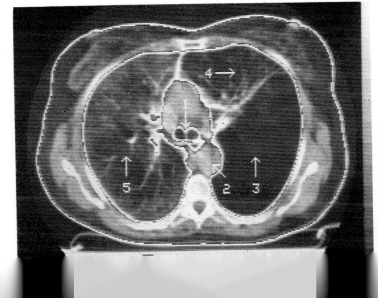

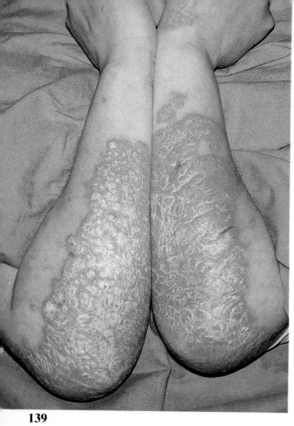

139

140

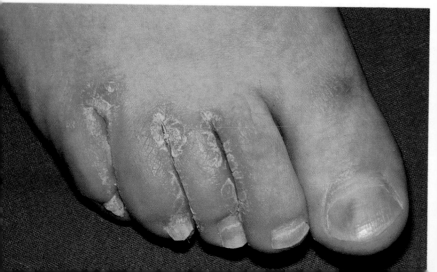

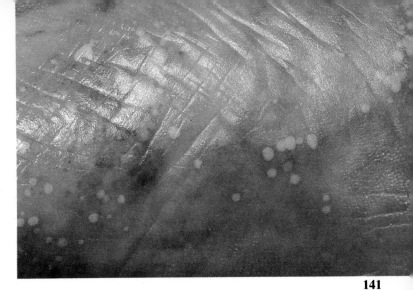

141

139, 140, 141 and 142 These patients all suffer from the same chronic skin disorder.
  a What skin disorder is this?
  b Name the morphological variety seen in each of these sites:
   i)   the forearms
   ii)   the sole of the foot
   iii) the dorsum of the foot
   iv) the trunk.

142

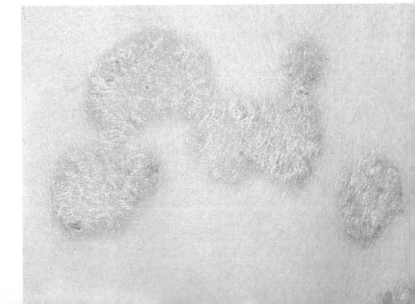

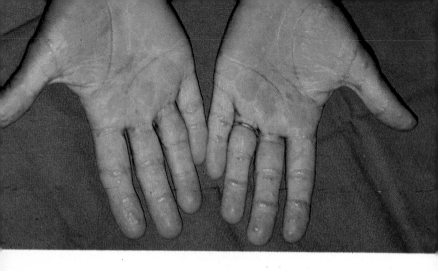

143 This forty year old woman complains of generalised pruritus and has
noticed pale stools and dark urine for some months. She is mildly
jaundiced.
a What are the lesions seen in the skin creases on her fingers?
b What is the likely diagnosis?
c Which serological test is most useful in establishing the diagnosis?

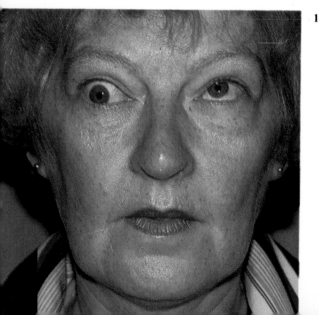

144 This patient is
attempting to look
upwards. Two years
ago non-surgical
treatment for an
endocrine disorder
was administered.
Following this
treatment the
appearance of her
eyes has worsened.
a What is the
diagnosis?
b What treatment
is she likely to
have had?
c What is likely to
be her current
endocrine status?

a What is the likely
diagnosis?
b How may the diagnosis
be confirmed?
c How should this
disorder be treated?

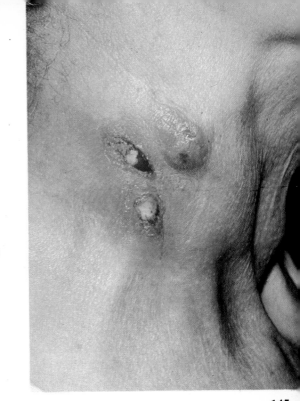

Since an attack of shingles
several months ago
(which produced a rash
on his palate only), this
patient has found
difficulty with some
movements of the left
arm. He has been asked
to shrug his shoulders.
a What two
abnormalities can be
seen?
b What is the
neurological lesion?

145

146

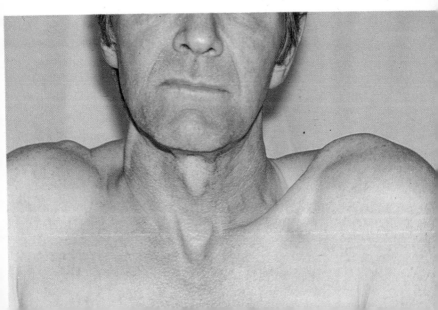

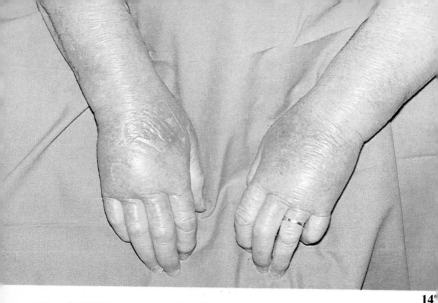

147 and 148 This woman has long history of productive cough. She recently complained of painful swollen wrists.
  a What is the diagnosis?
  b What may radiology of the hands and wrists show?
  c Which other diseases are associated with the hand and wrist disorder?

148

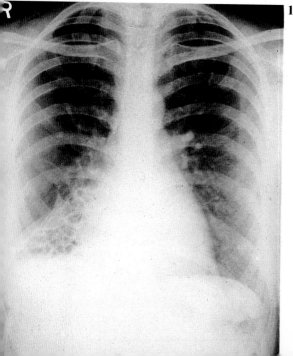

149 This man was admitted t[...] hospital following a convulsion and was note[...] to have widespread bruising. Blood glucose was 2.3 mmol/l. A 5% glucose infusion was commenced. His platele[...] count was 140 x 10^9/1, H[...] 13.1 g/dl, MCV 110 fl. The blood film showed round macrocytosis and stomatocytosis. Prothrombin time was prolonged at 60 seconds. The following day he became confused and developed ocular paresis and nystagmus.

149

What abnormality is present in addition to his bruising?
What are the two likeliest causes of his convulsion? What is the probable underlying etiology?
How should the bleeding disorder be corrected?
What is the cause of his deterioration and how could it have been prevented?

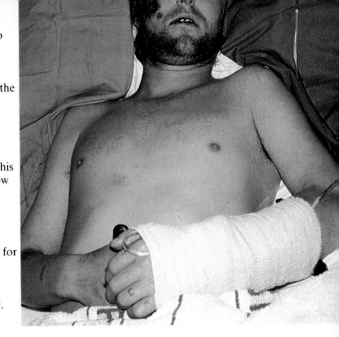

150

This child was referred for investigation of short stature and declining school performance. Bone age was retarded.
What are the radiological abnormalities?
What is the most likely diagnosis?
Is growth hormone therapy indicated?

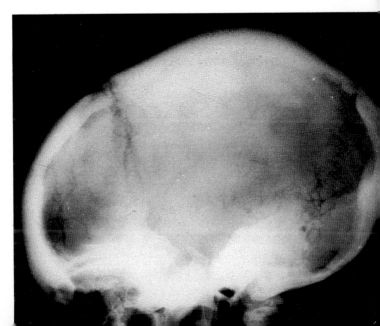

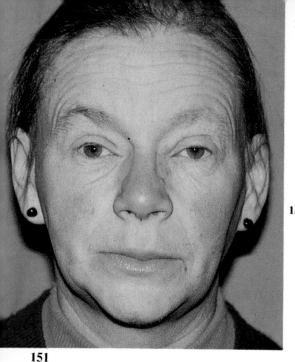

151

151 This patient complains of undue tiredness, dry skin and cold intolerance. Her skin appears to be becoming yellow.
  a What is the diagnosis?
  b Why is her skin becoming yellow?

152 This man has multiple myeloma. He complains of painful cold toes and fingers, especially in cold weather. His pedal pulses are normal.
  a What is the likely cause of this appearance?
  b What other cutaneous manifestations may occur?
  c What therapy is available?
  d What precautions should be taken when investigating this condition?

152

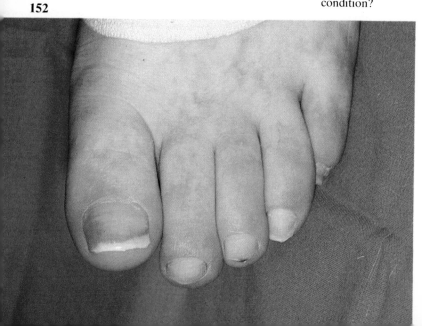

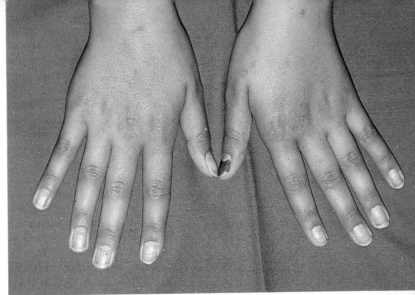

153

154

153 and 154 This patient complains of tiredness.
a What principal abnormality is seen in
 i) the hands?
 ii) the abdominal x-ray?
b What is the diagnosis, and what is the likely underlying cause in this case?

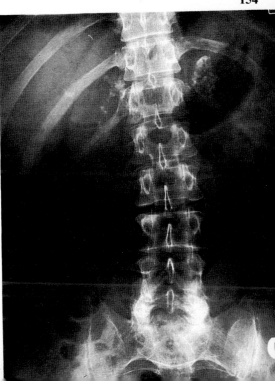

155 This patient with chronic compensated liver failure complained of increasingly painful abdominal distension and was admitted to hospital. A few days after admission he became mildly encephalopathic.
a What principal abnormality is seen here?
b What is likely to have precipitated his encephalopathy?
c List five other factors which may precipitate encephalopathy in these patients.

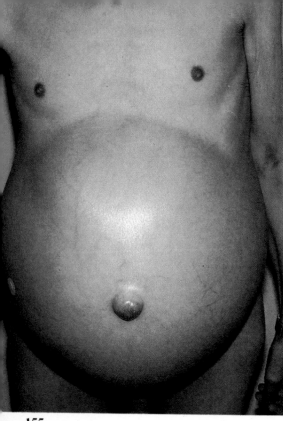

155

156

156 This man has multiple myeloma.
a What is this condition?
b Name three other disorders which may also predispose to this?

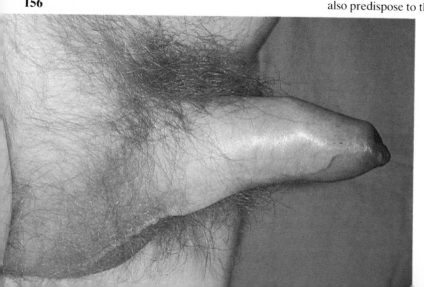

157 and 158 This patient suffers from a chronic gastrointestinal disorder. He has had recurrent scrotal lesions for years, and over the past few months has developed an enlarging skin lesion on the lower right chest wall.
a What name is given to the chest wall lesion?
b What is the underlying condition?

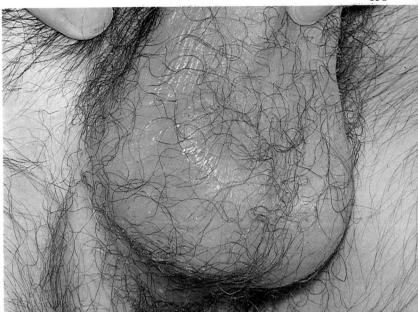

157

158

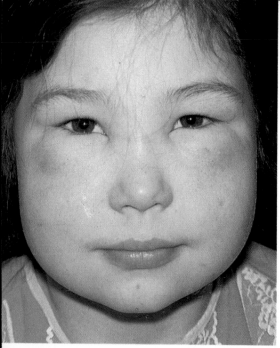

159

159 This young girl's serum calcium is low: she does not have clinical features of latent tetany.
  a What is the clinical diagnosis?
  b What is the most likely histological finding on biopsy of the appropriate organ?

160

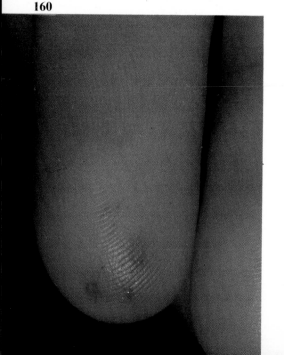

160 This patient presents with pyrexia.
  a What eponymous abnormality is shown here?
  b What is the likely diagnosis?
  c What other clues to this condition may be found on clinical examination?

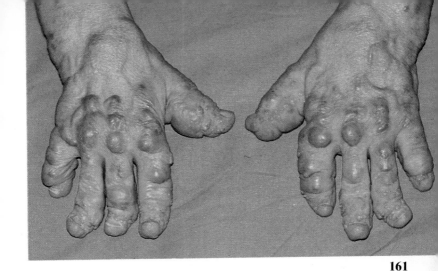

161

161 This patient complains of recurrent pain and swelling in all finger joints and both wrists. What two main differential diagnoses are suggested?

162

162 a What description is given to the individual lesions shown?
  b What is the diagnosis?
  c Which two infectious diseases are most commonly recognised as precipitants?

163 This woman is an insulin dependent diabetic.
a What is the diagnosis?
b Why is her pupil spared?

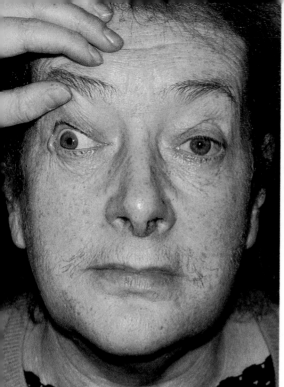

163

164 This patient feels as if she is walking 'on pebbles'.
a Of what condition is this foot deformity characteristic?
b What is the simplest means of relieving her symptoms?

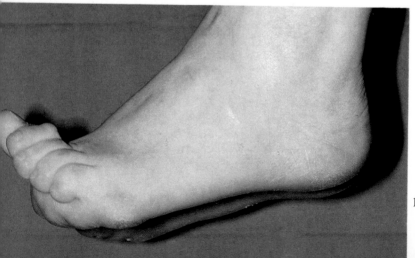

164

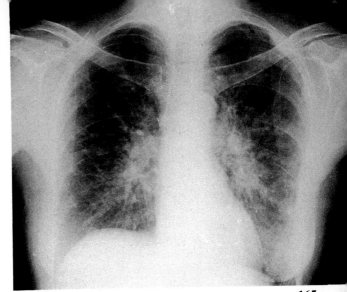

165

165 and 166 This patient complains of gradually progressive exertional dyspnoea.
  a What abnormalities are seen in the chest film?
  b What abnormalities are seen in the hand x-rays?
  c What is the diagnosis?

166

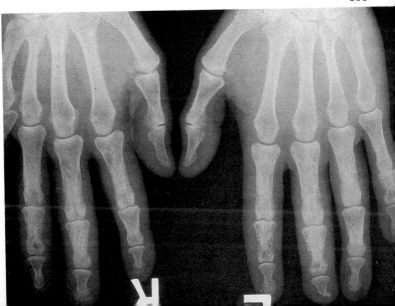

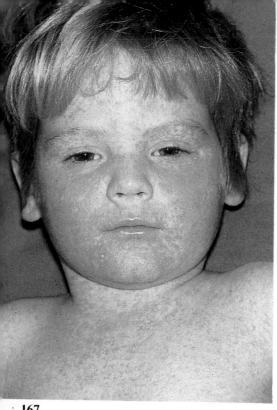

167 and 168 This boy
presented with right iliac
fossa pain. An
appendicectomy was
performed. He developed
this rash the following
day.
a What is the diagnosis?
b i) What are the oral
       lesions and
   ii) What is their
        significance?
c What may histology of
   the appendix show?

167

168

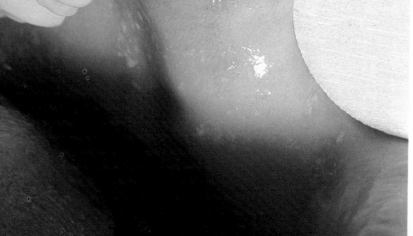

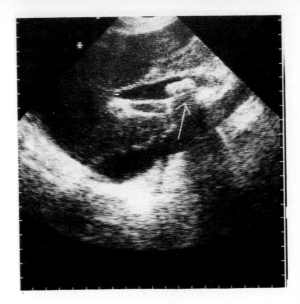

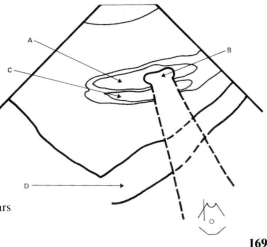

169 This fifty year old man who had a cholecystectomy six years ago now presents with jaundice, anorexia, nausea and vomiting.

    a Name the features labelled 'A', 'B', 'C' and 'D' shown on this para-sagittal scan of the upper abdomen.

    b List three other non-operative investigations which might be useful in demonstrating the biliary abnormality.

169

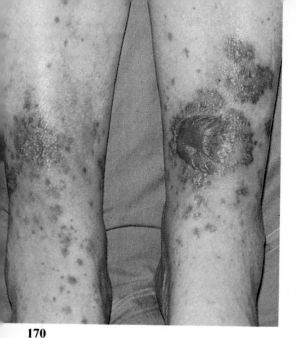

170

171

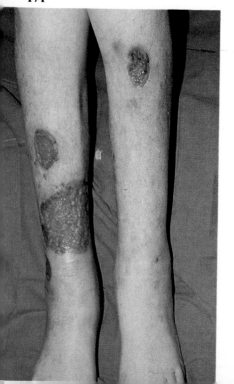

170 and 171 These patients both have rheumatoid arthritis.

a The lesions seen in both patients' lower legs have a common pathogenesis. What is it?

b List three other cutaneous manifestations of rheumatoid arthritis.

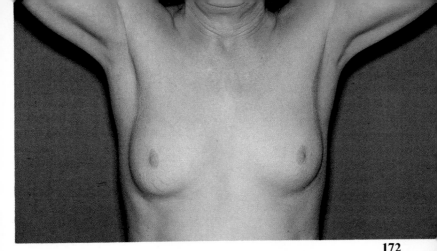

172

72 This patient's first and only pregnancy, twenty years ago, was complicated by retained placenta and prolonged post-partum haemorrhage.
   a What non-artefactual abnormality is seen here?
   b What is the likely diagnosis?
   c What are the usual early clinical features of this condition, following recovery from the precipitating illness?

173

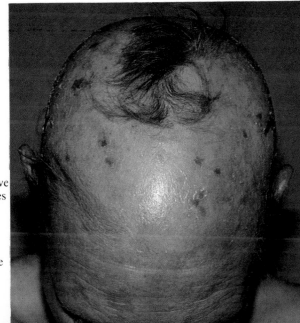

173 This patient has a positive serum Venereal Diseases Research Laboratories (VDRL) test.
   a What abnormality is seen in his scalp?
   b Suggest three possible diagnoses.

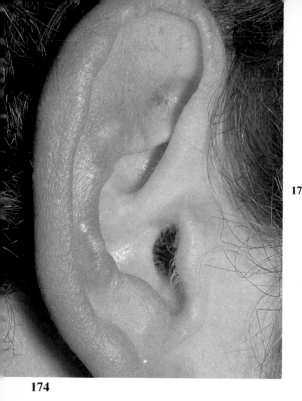

174

174 and 175 This patient has groups of lesions, similar to those seen on the ear and hand, on his feet and arms. He has no joint symptoms, but complains of recent weight loss and polydipsia.
a Of which non-infective skin condition are these appearances typical?
b Which metabolic disorder may be associated with this condition?

175

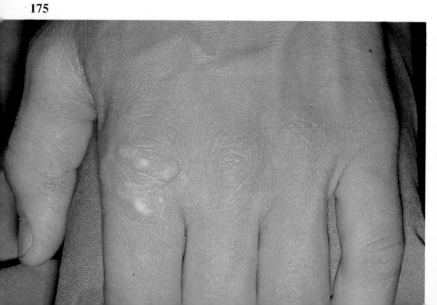

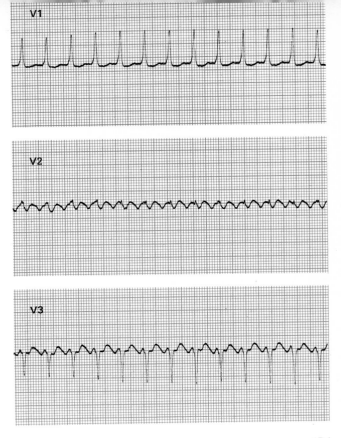

V1

V2

V3

176

176 This man complained of palpitations and a tachycardia of 150 beats per minute was noted.
a What is the dysrhythmia?
b What auscultatory finding may help differentiate this from paroxysmal atrial tachycardia?
c What are the effects of digoxin administration on this dysrhythmia?

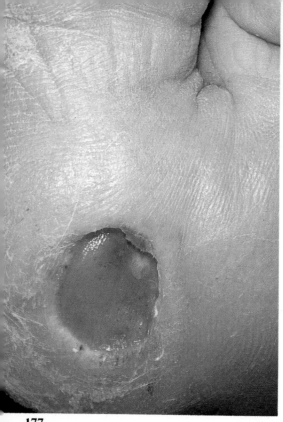

177

178

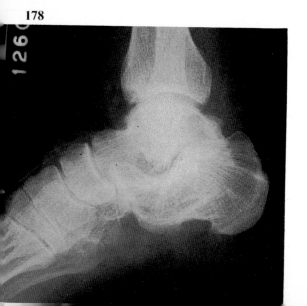

177 and 178

a What abnormalities are shown on this patient's foot and foot x-ray?

b What is the most likely diagnosis?

c Which organisms may be responsible?

179 This fifty-eight year old patient complains of back pain and stiffness, especially after periods of rest, of six months duration. The picture illustrates his full range of spinal flexion and extension. The distance from the sacrum to the twelfth dorsal vertebra varies four centimetres during this exercise. What is the most likely diagnosis?

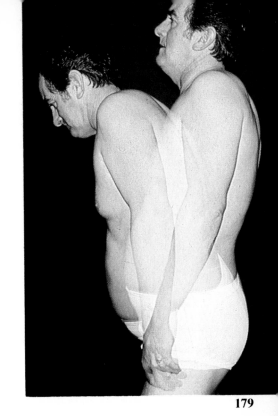

179

180

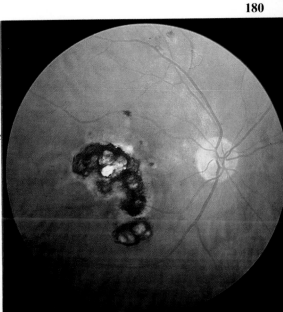

180 This woman has defective vision because of a lesion present since birth.
  a What abnormality of vision is likely?
  b What is the underlying cause?
  c Will her younger sister suffer from the same condition?

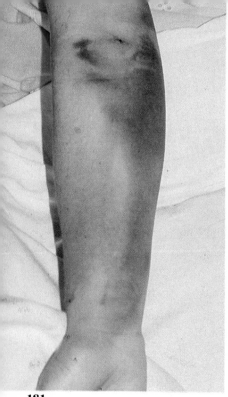

181

181 and 182 This patient complained of lethargy, pallor and increased bruising. She was noted to bleed excessively from venepuncture sites. Her haemoglobin was 8 g/dl, white cell count 178 x 10^9/1 and platelet count 21 x 10^9/1. Prothrombin time and partial thromboplastin time were prolonged, fibrinogen reduced, and fibrin degradation products present in excess.

a What underlying diagnosis does this blood film suggest?

b Which complication has occurred?

182

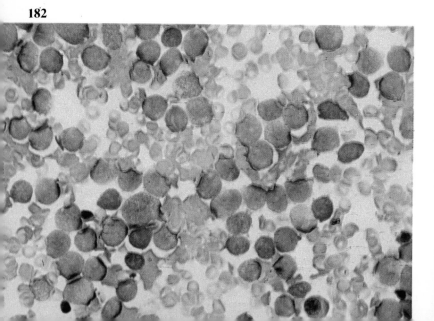

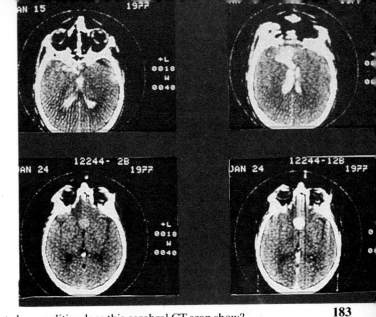

183 a What abnormalities does this cerebral CT scan show?

b What is the probable diagnosis?

183

184

184 This child was thought to be deaf by his parents. This appearance was present bilaterally.

a Describe the appearance and suggest the likely diagnosis.

b What abnormality should be detectable on testing hearing with a tuning fork?

c Are antibiotics indicated for this condition?

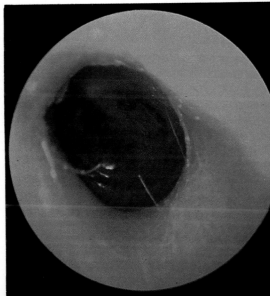

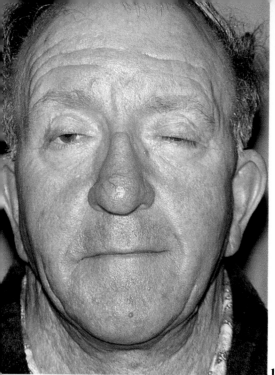

185 This sixty-two year old gardener has been unable to work because of increasing weakness, which progresses throughout the day. He has recently experienced several transient episodes of diplopia and of regurgitation of fluids down his nose.

a What ocular abnormality is shown?

b What is the likely diagnosis?

c How can this be confirmed simply?

d Is this age of onset unusual?

185

186 a What abnormality of the lips is shown?

b With what is this associated and what is the disease called?

c Is this condition associated with malignancy?

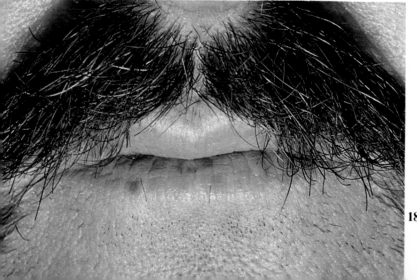

186

This thirty-two year old female patient complains of generalised pruritus. Examination reveals no dermatological abnormality.

a What abnormality is seen on chest x-ray?
b What is the likely diagnosis?
c What is the most likely histological variety in this case?

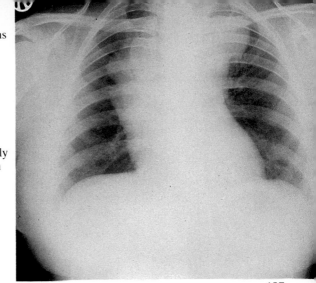

187

188

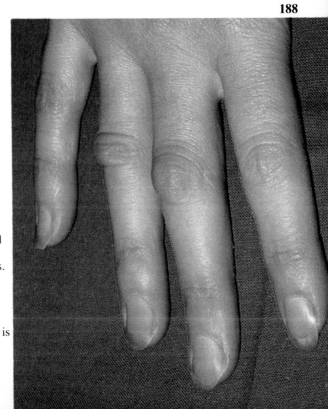

is woman complained out the unsightly pearance of her hands.
What abnormality is present?
How is the condition acquired?
With which condition is this associated?

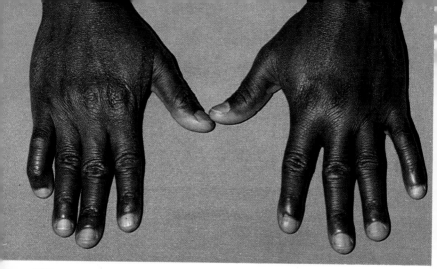

189

189 and 190 These two patients are suffering from the same condition. The
first complains of intense pain in the left hand of two days duration. The
second (whose hand x-ray is shown) has no symptoms.
a What principal abnormality is seen
  i)   in the hands?
  ii) in the x-rays?
b What is the most likely diagnosis, and what is the causative agent?
c What is the geographical distribution of this disorder?

190

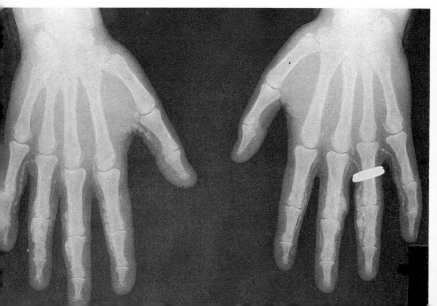

191 This patient was admitted to hospital after a major gastrointestinal bleed. The morning after admission this skin rash was seen to have developed. There is no history of similar rashes.
a What type of rash is this?
b Suggest two possible causes.

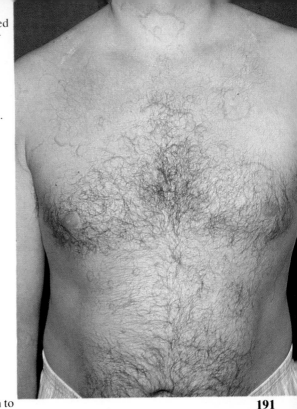

191

192 a What name is given to the ocular abnormality seen?
b Suggest two possible causes.

192

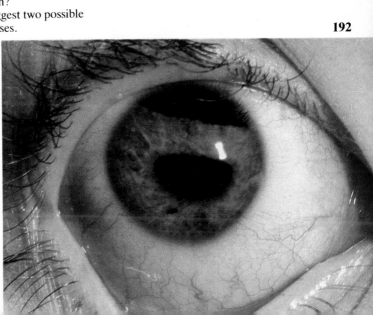

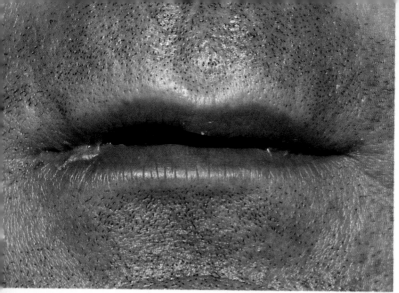

193

194

193 This man was seen two
hours after swallowing a
quantity of weed killer.
His appearance did not
change with oxygen
administration.
  a What abnormality is
     present and what is the
     likely cause?
  b What type of
     weedkiller has he
     taken?
  c What immediate
     treatment should be
     given?

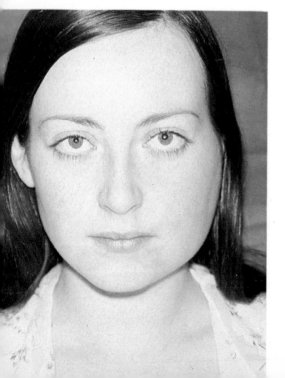

194 This patient was admitted
to hospital complaining of
headache, neck stiffness,
and drowsiness. The
following day this facial
appearance had
developed.
  a What is the likely
     diagnosis?
  b What would lumbar
     puncture show?
  c How is the diagnosis
     confirmed?

ANSWERS

The answers given below are necessarily brief as the aim of the series is to stimulate self-learning through further reading.

1 a A polypoid vascular tumour is invading the middle ear.
  b Glomus jugulare with involvement of the IXth, Xth and XIth cranial nerves.
  c Radiotherapy is often required when the tumour has caused extensive local destruction, but smaller tumours may be treated surgically.

2 a Leishman-Donovan bodies in a monocyte; visceral leishmaniasis.
  b Phlebotomus sandflies.
  c Pentavalent antimonials such as sodium stilbogluconate.

3 Rupture of the supraspinatus tendon.

4 a Prepatellar bursitis.
  b Housemaid's knee.
  c No. The prepatellar bursa does not communicate with the knee joint.

5 a Temporal (cranial, giant cell) arteritis. The symptoms are, however, not specific for this disorder.
  b i) Lingual and jaw claudication.
    ii) Raynaud's phenomenon of the tongue.
  c None. Tortuosity of the extracranial arteries is a normal finding at this age.

6 a Pressure sores.
  b Secondary amyloidosis, with renal glomerular involvement.
  c Rectal biopsy.

7 and 8
  a 'Rockerbottom' foot.
  b Trisomy 18. Edwards' syndrome.
  c Poor. Few children survive into their second year.
    (Average male survival is under sixty days. Females tend to survive longer).

9 a These represent pericardial fluid.
  b i) Variable opening of the mitral valve.
    ii) Early collapse in systole of the right ventricular outflow tract.
      These are signs of cardiac tamponade.
  c Pericardiocentesis. This is a relatively simple procedure under ultrasonic control.

10 a Strawberry naevus (angiomatous naevus, cavernous naevus/haemangioma).

    b i)   Failure to resolve spontaneously (cosmetic).

        ii)   Ulceration.

        iii)   Feeding difficulty.

        iv)   Haemorrhage.

11 a Herpetic whitlows.

    b Electron microscopy of aspirated blister fluid.

12 a Ichthyosis.

    b Hodgkin's disease.

    c i)   Other malignancies — lymphosarcoma, mycosis fungoides, Kaposi's sarcoma.

        ii)   Leprosy.

        iii)   Malnutrition — especially vitamin A deficiency.

13 a Argyll Robertson pupil

    b False.

      The Argyll Robertson pupil of neurosyphilis is characteristically small. A dilated pupil which reacts as described may be found in association with pineal tumours, diabetes mellitus and brainstem encephalitis.

14 a Hypermetropia.

    b Pseudopapilloedema (may be a normal feature of the hypermetropic fundus).

15 a Aplastic anaemia.

    b Absence of lymphadenopathy or hepatosplenomegaly which would suggest an alternative cause of pancytopaenia.

    c The marrow is hypoplastic with extensive fatty replacement.

    d Sulphamethoxazole.

16, 17 and 18

    a Multiple discrete lytic lesions in the skull. Lytic lesions of the lumbar vertebral bodies. Compression fracture of the body of the twelfth thoracic vertebral body.

    b Hyperviscosity syndrome due to polymerisation of the excessive immunoglobulin and/or thrombocytopaenia and anaemia due to marrow failure.

    c Serum creatinine, blood urea, haemoglobin, and serum albumin.

19 and 20

    a i)   Left Horner's syndrome.

        ii)   Wasting of first dorsal interosseus muscle on both sides; multiple healed scars, mostly of the right hand, claw hand on the right.

    b i)   Syringomyelia.

        ii)   Intrinsic tumour of the cervical spinal cord (eg ependymoma, glioma).

            Bilateral lower brachial plexus lesions (eg in association with Pancoast tumours) unlikely.

21 a Proptosis (this patient may also have exophthalmos — sclera visible between the iris and lower lid — but this is best seen from the front).

b Exophthalmometer — measuring the distance between the lateral angle of the orbit and an imaginary line perpendicular to the cornea's anterior surface.

22 a i) Striae (old).

ii) Widening of the primary areola.

iii) Montgomery's tubercles.

iv) Dilated superficial veins.

b Pregnancy.

c Between eight and twelve weeks ago. (Darkening of the primary areola, and development of the secondary areola, which occur from twelve and sixteen weeks onwards respectively, are not yet seen).

23 and 24

Hyperuricaemia — the first patient has tophaceous gout, the second patient has psoriasis.

(Severe exfoliative psoriasis with rapid epidermal cell division may lead to hyperuricaemia due to increased turnover of purines).

25 a Sinus tachycardia; P mitrale; anteroseptal myocardial infarction; ST elevation in leads V1 — 4.

b He has developed a ventricular aneurysm. The P mitrale may indicate mitral regurgitation and dilatation of the left atrium.

c A diffuse, often laterally displaced apex beat with a double or paradoxical impulse is characteristic of ventricular aneurysm; the murmur of mitral regurgitation may be present.

26 and 27

a i) Irregular grey-brown discolouration.

ii) Expansion of the lower end of the femur. (The Ehrlenmayer flask deformity).

b Gaucher's disease.

c Massive splenomegaly, hepatomegaly.

d Raised serum acid phosphatase (of bony origin).

28 a Swelling over front and left lateral aspect of neck.

b i) Isotopic thyroid scan.

ii) Ultrasonic scan of thyroid.

iii) Fine needle — aspiration biopsy.

iv) (Serum thyroxine and tri-iodothyronine levels).

v) (Serum thyroid antibodies).

c i) Colloid cyst of thyroid.

ii) Thyroid adenoma.

iii) Thyroid carcinoma.

29 a He has developed an inhibitor to factor VIII.

b Haemophiliac or von Willebrand patients transfused with factor VIII; post partum women; autoimmune diseases (e.g. systemic lupus erythematosus); drug reactions.

30 a Rheumatoid nodules.
   b Extensor aspect forearm, olecranon (as shown), sacrum, achilles tendon, extensor and flexor tendons in the hand; sclerae, myocardium, lung.
   c The presence of nodules is typically associated with seropositive and more aggressive rheumatoid arthritis.

31 a Malignant melanomata.
   b i) Surgery — wide excision + split skin grafting (from the unaffected limb) + (where practical) dissection of draining nodes.
      ii) Chemotherapy
         — systemic: single (eg. Dacarbazine) or combined regimes.
         — regional perfusion (eg. phenylalanine mustard).
      iii) Radiotherapy (especially for malignant change in Hutchinson's lentigo).
      iv) Immunotherapy — BCG,
                        Vaccinia, corynebacterium parvum.
      v) Hyperthermia.

32 a Short stature; infantile proportions — i.e. in ratio of trunk to limb; coarse facial features.
   b Juvenile hypothyroidism.
   c Measurement of serum thyroxine and thyroid stimulating hormone concentrations.

33 a Psoriasis.
   b Nail changes include   i) pitting
                        ii) onycholysis
                        iii) discoloration
                        iv) thickening.

34 and 35
   a No, intelligence is not affected.
   b The reflexes are often impaired with the exception of the ankle jerks.
   c No. It should be normal.

36 a Basal cell carcinoma (rodent ulcer). Squamous carcinoma is much less likely.
   b Conjunctival keratinisation and chronic keratitis. Inadequate radiation may induce metaplasia to squamous carcinoma.
   c i) Surgical excision.
      ii) Cryotherapy.
      iii) Topical cytotoxic drugs such as 5-fluorouracil.

37 a The ulnar nerve.
   b There is wasting of the thenar eminence.
   c Either the ulnar nerve is supplying all the intrinsic muscles of the hand as it does in 2-3% of the population or the lesion is in the brachial plexus damaging the lower trunk.

38 Hydrochlorothiazide, chlorpropamide. (This is a photosensitive eruption).

39 a Lacework expansion of the marrow cavities with loss of the normal fine medullary trabeculation particularly in the phalanges.
b Thalassaemia major.
c Splenectomy (following which the peripheral platelet, white cell and nucleated red cell counts rise).
d Pneumococcal infection.

40 a Sebaceous naevus.
b Malignant transformation may occur (eg. basal cell carcinoma in approximately 20%).

41 a Brushfield's spots, around the iris.
b Down's syndrome (trisomy 21).

42 a Looser's zones (pseudo fractures).
b Osteomalacia.
c Osteomalacia is well-recognised association of treatment with
   i) Phenytoin.
   ii) Phenobarbitone.
   iii) Primidone.
   iv) Other enzyme inducer drugs.
   (Limited exposure to sunlight may contribute).

43 a Sunlight — these are solar keratoses.
b These may be premalignant — Squamous carcinoma may develop.

44 Artefact
(These are 'pinch' skin graft donor sites).

45 a Pyogenic granuloma.
b Capillary proliferation.

46 and 47
a Increased anteroposterior diameter ('barrel' chest).
b Atopic eczema (which more typically affects the flexures).
c i) Conjunctivitis.
   ii) Atopic cataract.
   iii) Keratoconus (conical cornea).

48 a 'Hair on end' appearance.
b Extramedullary haemopoiesis/expanded marrow cavity.
c Thalassaemia major.

49 a Tinea incognito.
b Steroid-modified ringworm infection.

50 a Ambiguous external genitalia with clitoromegaly and fusion of the labia.

b Congenital adrenal hyperplasia of the salt-losing type.
c 21-hydroxylase deficiency.

51 a Ascites, hepatomegaly and, less commonly, splenomegaly.
  b Pulsus paradoxus.
  c The jugular venous pressure is characteristically raised and rises further on inspiration (Kussmaul's sign).
  d Excision of the pericardium is the treatment of choice, in addition to the standard treatment of congestive cardiac failure.

52 and 53
  a i) Swelling and erythema suggesting acute arthritis.
    ii) Erythematous, scaling, pustular eruption.
  b Gonococcal arthritis and dermatitis; anorectal gonorrhoea is the likely site of infection.
  c Culture of urine, blood, synovial fluid, rectal and urethral; smears and skin lesions.

54 a 1 in 4 (Autosomal dominant inheritance).
  b At present there is no reliable method of detecting Huntington's chorea prior to the onset of symptoms.
  c None. (Although cholestatic hepatitis associated with phenothiazine therapy may occur).

55 a Multiple shallow aphthous ulcers on reddened bases on the tongue, and several vesicles (pustules) on the thumb.
  b Primary herpes simplex — acute herpetic gingivostomatitis and herpetic whitlows.
  c Thumb-sucking.

56 a Hepatic bruit.
  b Hepatocellular carcinoma.
  c i) Cirrhosis (especially haemochromatosis, can occur in any type).
    ii) Hepatitis B infection.
    iii) Aflatoxin (produced by aspergillus flavus).
    iv) Oral contraceptive (very rarely).

57 a Adult coeliac disease (gluten-sensitive enteropathy).
  b i) Iron deficiency, secondary to malabsorption.
    ii) Hyposplenism — splenic atrophy.
  c i) Small bowel lymphoma.
    ii) Ulcerative jejunoileitis.

58 a Achondroplasia.
  b Endochondral ossification.
  c Increasing paternal age.

59 a Bilateral hilar and mediastinal lymphadenopathy.
  b The linear lucency separating hilar from mediastinal nodes indicates that the nodes are discrete, and therefore more likely to be benign.

60 and 61

    a Gouty tophi.

    b Central nervous system.

    c i)   Uric acid nephrolithiasis.

        ii) Uric acid nephropathy.

        iii) Hypertensive renal disease.

62 a i)   'Hound dog' facial expression.

        ii) Masseter, temporalis and sternomastoid wasting.

        iii) Frontal balding.

    b Myotonic dystrophy.

63 a Osgood Schlatter's disease.

       (Osteochondritis of the tibial tuberosity.)

64 a Increased pigmentation and presence of buccal pigmentation.

    b Adrenal insufficiency.

    c i)   Plasma cortisol and response to tetracosactrin — low cortisol and diminished response.

        ii) Plasma adrenocorticotrophic hormone — greatly elevated.

    d i)   Autoimmune disease of adrenal gland.

        ii) Tuberculosis.

        iii) Metastatic carcinoma.

        iv) Adrenalectomy.

        v) Systemic fungal infections.

        vi) Amyloidosis.

65 Adenocarcinoma (especially gastric). The illustration shows axillary acanthosis nigricans.

66 a Erythema ab igne.

    b Prolonged application of heat (via hot water bottle, poultices) for pain relief.

67 a Corneal arcus.

    b It suggests underlying hypercholesterolaemia; a potentially treatable risk factor in ischaemic heart disease.

68 a Surgical emphysema (note the dressing of a left upper intercostal drain).

    b Pleural aspiration/biopsy.

69 a Healed digital infarcts.

    b Rheumatoid arthritis.

    c Mononeuritis multiplex.

       (Early peripheral neuropathy is possible; secondary to vasculitic involvement of vasa nervorum).

70 i)   Spironolactone.

      ii) Digitalis (possibly, digoxin).

iii) Oestrogens eg. stilboestrol.
iv) Isoniazid.
v) Ethionamide.
vi) Griseofulvin.
vii) Testosterone.
viii) Cimetidine.

71 a Loss of the prosthetic valve sounds and the development of the murmur of aortic regurgitation.
b Complete heart block due to damage to the conducting system during valve replacement.
c A permanent transvenous ventricular pacemaker was inserted.

72 a Leukoplakia. Intraepithelial/squamous carcinoma must be excluded by histology.
b i) Tobacco smoking.
ii) Local irritation — ill fitting dentures, dental caries.
iii) Candida albicans infection.
iv) Severe iron deficiency anaemia.

73 and 74
a Wasting of the small hand muscles (most noticeably 1st dorsal interosseus) on left.
b i) Opacity left apex.
ii) Destruction of proximal end of 2nd left rib.
c Apical bronchogenic carcinoma (Pancoast tumour), with intercostal and brachial plexus nerve invasion.

75 a Purpuric rash.
b Mononeuritis multiplex (possibly early sensorimotor polyneuropathy).
c Polyarteritis nodosa.
d i) Leucocytosis.
ii) Raised ESR.
iii) Positive hepatitis B surface antigen.

76 a i) Violaceous discolouration of skin of left cheek.
ii) Depressed nasal bridge (a result of granulomatous destruction of the anterior nasal septum).
b i) Sarcoidosis.
ii) Tuberculosis.
c Mantoux test.

77 a Delayed relaxation phase of the ankle jerk.
b The serum thyroid stimulating hormone (TSH) level.

78 a Group A beta haemolytic streptococcal infection.
b i) Acute rheumatic fever.
ii) Acute glomerulonephritis (typically diffuse proliferative type).

79 a Inferior wall aneurysm.
b Changes of full-thickness inferior/true posterior myocardial infarction:

Q waves in standard leads II, III, AVF, dominant R waves in the right-sided chest leads; persistent ST elevation in leads II, III and AVF; ST depression in the right sided chest leads.

  c The murmur of mitral incompetence may be heard if disruption to the posterior leaflet of the mitral valve has occurred.

80 a Koilonychia (spoon-shaped nails).
    b i) Oesophageal web (Plummer-Vinson/Paterson-Kelly syndromes) in association with iron deficiency.
      ii) Chronic blood loss from peptic or neoplastic oesophageal disease. (Oesophageal web itself predisposes to oesophageal carcinoma).

81 a Splenomegaly.
    b Splenomegaly makes 'idiopathic' thrombocytopenic purpura (ITP) very unlikely; and lymphoma, leukaemia, hypersplenism likely.
    c Normal. Megakaryocyte numbers may be increased. In ITP, thrombocytopenia follows peripheral autoimmune destruction of platelets.

82 a Herpes zoster ophthalmicus.
    b i) Conjunctivitis, keratitis, iridocyclitis, optic neuritis (rarely).
      ii) Encephalomyelitis.
      iii) Associated cranial nerve involvement (especially VIIth with facial palsy).
      iv) Secondary streptococcal/staphylococcal infection.
      v) Haemorrhagic zoster (purpura fulminans).
      vi) Dissemination (immunosuppressed patients).
      vii) Post-herpetic neuralgia.

83 a Microaneurysms, dot and blot haemorrhages, hard exudates. Maculopathy.
    b Diabetes mellitus.

84 and 85
    a i) Striae.
      ii) Diffuse hyperpigmentation.
    b Right oculomotor (third cranial nerve) palsy.
    c Nelson's syndrome. (Pituitary corticotroph adenoma showing progressive growth after bilateral adrenalectomy for Cushing's disease. These tumours are often locally invasive).

86 a In most patients the abnormal cells are B lymphocytes but T-cell CLL may infrequently occur.
    b i) Hypogammaglobulinaemia.
      ii) Monoclonal gammopathy.
    c i) Bone marrow failure.
      ii) Autoimmune haemolytic anaemia.
    d None; there is no characteristic chromosomal abnormality.

87 a i) Heberden's nodes.
  ii) Bouchard's nodes.
 b Osteophytes.
  (Occasionally joint effusions and painful cystic swelling adjacent to the joints may accompany rapidly developing Heberden's and Bouchard's nodes).

88 a Turner's syndrome.
 b Features of aortic coarctation include,
  i) Systemic hypertension.
  ii) Inequality of radial pulses and of blood pressure in the arms (if the coarctation is proximal to the left subclavian artery — most are not).
  iii) Radiofemoral delay.
  iv) Scapular collateral vessels, with or without bruits.
  v) Systolic murmur over the left upper chest (front and back).
  vi) Systolic murmur from frequently associated bicuspid aortic valve.
  vii) Left ventricular hypertrophy.

89 i) Fracture of the waist of the scaphoid.
  ii) Bone density relatively greater in the scaphoid, suggesting avascular necrosis.

90 a i) Skin nodules.
  ii) Café au lait patch.
  iii) Axillary freckling (Crowe's sign).
 b Neurofibromatosis (Von Recklinghausen's disease) — axillary freckling is said to be pathognomonic.

91 a Ringworm: spreading tinea cruris. Likely infecting organism tinea rubrum.
 b Griseofulvin (orally).

92 a Skull base fracture involving the orbit with an expanding intracerebral (probably extradural) haematoma.
 b Skull x-rays may demonstrate the fracture. Cerebral CT scan is the investigation of choice followed by neurosurgical intervention. "Blind" evacuation may be necessary if CT scanning is not available immediately.

93 a Prepatellar bursitis (housemaid's knee).
 b None. It is a sterile inflammation due to trauma.

94 a Family history; predominantly proximal muscle weakness; absence of bulbar damage; absence of pyramidal signs.
 b Physiotherapy. Swimming is particularly beneficial.

95 a A ganglion.
 b Fibrous tissue of the joint capsule or tendon sheath.
 c Traumatic obliteration (eg sharp blow) is associated with a high rate of recurrence. Excision is more likely to be successful.

96 and 97

    a Tuberous sclerosis (epiloia); adenoma sebaceum.

    b Leaf-shaped pale macules (a larger macule adjacent to the umbilicus, smaller lesions along the costal margins).

    c Nodules of glial proliferation usually on the surface of the cerebral cortex, gyri and ventricular surfaces.

    d i) Shagreen patch.

       ii) Subungual fibroma

    (Café au lait spots, and pedunculated fibromata may also be found but are less typical).

98 a Left sided calcified pleural plaque.

    b Asbestos exposure (although pleural calcification can develop following any inflammatory pleural disease — e.g. empyema).

    c i) Pulmonary fibrosis.

       ii) Bronchial carcinoma.

       iii) Pleural mesothelioma.

99 a Erythema ab igne.

    b Infra red radiation.

    c Yes. Epitheliomatous change has been described.

    d Hypothyroidism.

100 a Coloboma.

    b Congenital — defective closure of embryonic cleft.

    c May be associated with colobomata (of varying extent) of anterior uvea and adjacent retina.

101 a Pretibial myxoedema.

    b Graves' disease.

    c Corticosteroids i) under occlusive plastic dressing.

                     ii) injected intralesionally.

102 a Pityriasis versicolor.

    b Fungal infection — *pityrosoporum* species.

    c i) Demonstration of yeasts and mycelia in scrapings.

       ii) Pale yellow fluorescence under Wood's light.

103 a Herpes labialis (cold sores).

    b Herpes simplex virus type 1.

    c Commonly associated with underlying bacterial infection

       eg. lobar pneumonia

          bacterial meningitis.

104 a Autosomal dominant.

    b Epilepsy.

105 and 106

    a Violaceous flat-topped polygonal papules.

    b Lichen planus.

    c Epitheliomatous transformation may occur in ulcerative mouth
      lesions.

107 Blindness in his left eye due to ischaemic optic atrophy. Cholesterol
    crystals and mural plaques can be seen in the upper nasal quadrant.

108 a Herpes zoster ophthalmicus.
    b It indicates that the cornea and uveal tract may be involved.
    c Acyclovir, vidarabine, or idoxuridine will limit viral replication.
      Systemic corticosteroids may reduce the incidence of post herpetic
      neuralgia but are contraindicated in the immunocompromised host.
      Local corticosteroids and atropine may be useful if anteror uveitis has
      developed.

109 a i)   Extensive soft tissue calcification.
      ii)   Cardiomegaly.
    b Dermatomyositis.

110 a Urticaria pigmentosa.
    b Abnormal proliferation of mast cells.
    c Mast cell degranulation, with release of vasoactive peptides
      (histamine, kinins).
    d Codeine phosphate, alcohol (also salicyclic acid, polymixin B).

111 a Keratoacanthoma.
    b Squamous carcinoma.

112 and 113
    a i)   Perianal disease — fistulae, fissures, skin tags.
      ii)   Erythema nodosum.
    b Crohn's disease.
    c i)   Ulcerative colitis.
      ii)   Yersinia, salmonella, campylobacter enteritides.
      iii) Tuberculosis.
      iv) Sarcoidosis (liver, salivary glands may be affected).

114 a Pruritus.
    b Cholestyramine.

115 a Pigment disturbance and exudation adjacent to and encroaching on
      the macula.
    b Senile macular degeneration.
    c Choroid.

116 a Swelling behind left sternomastoid.
    b Left Horner's syndrome secondary to cervical mass.
    c She has developed gastric carcinoma as a complication of long-
      standing pernicious anaemia, with resultant cervical
      lymphadenopathy (Troisier's sign).

17 a Ehlers Danlos syndrome
   b i) Skin hyperelasticity.
     ii) Skin and blood vessel fragility. (Easy bruising and delayed skin
          healing with papyraceous scars and molluscoid pseudotumours.)
     iii) Joint hyperextensibility — flat feet, genu recurvatum,
          kyphoscoliosis.
     iv) Characteristic facies — wide nasal bridge, hypertelorism,
          epicanthic folds.
     v)   Occasionally, retinal angioid streaks, blue sclerae, aortic
          dissection.

18 a Beau's line.
   b When isolated to one nail, local injury is the likely cause. When all
     nails are affected, these indicate recent systemic illness interfering
     with nail growth temporarily (eg. measles, mumps, pneumonia,
     coronary thrombosis).

19 a Sabre tibiae.
   b i) Paget's disease.
     ii) Congenital syphilis.
   c Osteogenic sarcoma, complicating Paget's disease.

20 and 121
   a Arachnodactyly.
   b Subluxation of the lens (upwards).
   c Marfan's syndrome: autosomal dominant.
   d Homocystinuria (in this condition the lens is said typically to sublux
     downwards).

22 a Palmar erythema.
   b i) Cirrhosis (especially alcoholic).
     ii) Normal pregnancy.
     iii) Rheumatoid arthritis.
     iv) Thyrotoxicosis.
     v)   Dermatological disorders — eczema, psoriasis, pityriasis rubra
          pilaris.
          Others include polycythaemia, diabetes mellitus, mitral valve
          disease, beri-beri. May occasionally be inherited.

23 Post-herpetic neuralgia.

24 and 125
   a Calcaneal spurs.
   b Reiter's disease.

26 a Band keratopathy.
   b Parathyroid exploration/parathyroidectomy.

27 a i) Infected branchial cyst.
     ii) Tuberculous lymphadenopathy/abscess.
   b i) Clinical: infected branchial cyst tends to cause sternomastoid

spasm. Tuberculosis tends to cause fixation to the overlying tissues.

    ii) Aspiration, microscopy, culture (+ additional evidence of tuberculosis: Mantoux, chest x-ray).

128 a 'Senile' cataract.
    b Diabetes mellitus.
    c These include:
      i)   Refractory disturbances — hypermetropia with rising blood glucose; myopia with falling blood glucose.
      ii)   Rubeosis iridis.
      iii) Retinopathy — background, proliferative.
      iv) Intrinsic and extrinsic ocular muscle paralysis (cranial nerve lesions and autonomic neuropathy).

129 a i)   Type II diabetes mellitus.
      ii)   Mental retardation.
      iii) Hypogonadism.
      iv) Muscle hypotonia.
    b i)   Laurence-Moon-Biedl syndrome (polydactyly, retinitis pigmentosa).
      ii)   Alstrom syndrome (nerve deafness).
      iii) Biemond syndrome (polydactyly, iris colobomata).

130 a Complete heart block with a high nodal escape rhythm. The QRS complex is normal.
    b Congenital.
    c His bundle electrocardiography.
    d None.

131 a Papilloedema with peripapillary flame haemorrhages.
    b Acute mountain sickness leading to cerebral oedema.
    c Immediate descent. Delay may be fatal.

132 a Thyroglossal cyst.
    b None; it arises from a downgrowth of endoderm in the midline.

133 a Oval macrocytes; hypersegmented polymorphonuclear leukocytes.
    b Subacute degeneration of the spinal cord due to vitamin B12 deficiency.
    c Optic atrophy; spastic paraplegia; mental changes including depression, dementia, confusional psychosis; peripheral neuropathy.

134 a i)   Right ptosis.
      ii)   Right miosis.
      iii) Sutured laceration overlying sternomastoid and the right anterior triangle.
    b Horner's syndrome due to damage to the cervical sympathetic fibres.

135 a i)   Intrinsic muscle wasting (most noticeably of first dorsal interossei).

ii) Prominent ulnar styloids.

iii) Prominent metacarpal heads.

iv) Ulnar deviation at the metacarpophalangeal joints (especially of left hand).

v) 'Z' deformity of left thumb.

b Rheumatoid arthritis.

c Rupture of the extensor digitorum tendons (third, fourth, fifth).

136 a There are bilateral nodular opacities, most marked in the lower and mid zones.

b i) Pulmonary function tests may show a restrictive ventilatory defect with reduced transfer factor, hypoxaemia and hypocapnia.

ii) Precipitating antibodies to avian protein may be detected.

iii) Provocation testing may reproduce the symptoms and support the diagnosis.

c Examples include: farmer's lung; bagassosis (sugar cane); byssinosis (cotton); cheese washer's lung; coffee worker's lung; detergent worker's lung; maltworker's lung; maple-bark worker's lung; mushroom worker's lung; prawnworker's lung; suberosis (cork); woodworker's lung.

137 This includes

i) Femoral hernia.

ii) Ectopic testis.

iii) Femoral lymphadenopathy.

iv) Saphena varix.

v) Psoas abscess.

vi) Femoral aneurysm.

138 1 Carina with right and left main bronchi.

2 Descending thoracic aorta.

3 Bulla in left lung.

4 Normal left lung parenchyma.

5 Normal right lung with small emphysematous bullae throughout the parenchyma.

139, 140, 141 and 142

a Psoriasis.

b i) Elephantine ('psoriasis inveterata').

ii) Flexural/intertriginous.

iii) Pustular.

iv) Nummular (the commonest form).

143 a Xanthomata.

b Primary biliary cirrhosis.

c Antimitochondrial antibody (A.M.A.). Presence of A.M.A. makes extrahepatic biliary obstruction unlikely.

144 a Ophthalmic Graves' disease.

Upward gaze is most typically impaired in this condition, owing to oedema and to lymphocytic and fatty infiltration of the orbital

contents, particularly of the extra ocular muscles.
  b Radioactive iodine.
  c Infiltrative eye disease may occur irrespective of thyroid status.
     Post-radioactive iodine hypothyroidism, however, is most likely to
     induce progressive eye changes.

145 a Scrofula — tuberculous cervical lymphadenitis.
  b i)   Biopsy — histological evidence of tuberculosis.
     ii) Bacteriological culture — but isolation rate of mycobacterium
          tuberculosis is only about 60%.
  c Anti-tuberculosis chemotherapy.
     eg. Rifampicin.
         Ethambutol.
         Isoniazid.

146 a i)   Wasting of left sternomastoid.
     ii) Loss of action of left trapezius.
  b Left XIth cranial (accessory) nerve paralysis.

147 and 148
  a Bronchiectasis with hypertrophic pulmonary osteoarthropathy.
  b Periosteal elevation with new bone formation.
  c Primary intrathoracic malignancy is the commonest association.
     Other causes include lung abscess, empyema, cyanotic congenital
     heart disease, cirrhosis and inflammatory bowel disease.

149 a Jaundice.
  b Hypoglycaemia or alcohol withdrawal if the patient was alcoholic.
  c Fresh frozen plasma will be more effective than vitamin K.
  d The ocular signs suggest Wernicke's encephalopathy rather than
     delirium tremens or hepatic encephalopathy, and may have been
     precipitated by the glucose infusion. Thiamine should have been given
     beforehand.

150 a Widening of the sutures; multiple sutural (Wormian) bones.
  b Hypothyroidism.
  c No.

151 a Hypothyroidism.
  b She is hypercarotenaemic (incidentally she was found to have an
     associated vitamin B_{12} deficiency).

152 a He has developed cryoglobulinaemia.
  b Raynaud's phenomenon; livedo reticularis; digital ulceration.
  c Protection of the extremities from cold; specific treatment of the
     underlying myeloma; plasmapheresis is of particular benefit if the
     cryoglobulin is IgM.
  d Blood should be taken and maintained at 37° to allow the detection of
     cryoglobulins.

153 and 154
- a i) Knuckle pigmentation.
  - ii) Adrenal calcification.
- b Primary adrenal insufficiency; tuberculosis.

155 a Ascites.
- b Paracentesis.
- c i) Alcohol.
  - ii) Drugs — e.g. diuretics, narcotics.
  - iii) Gastrointestinal haemorrhage.
  - iv) Infection.
  - v) Surgery (especially portacaval shunting).

156 a Priapism.
- b i) Chronic granulocytic leukaemia.
  - ii) Spinal cord injury.
  - iii) Sickle-cell anaemia.

157 and 158
- a Pyoderma gangrenosum
- b Ulcerative colitis.

159 a Nephrotic syndrome. Her serum calcium, corrected for hypoalbuminaemia, is normal.
- b 'Minimal change' nephropathy, on renal biopsy.

160 a Osler's nodes (tender; appear typically in finger and toe pulps, thenar and hypothenar eminences).
- b Infective endocarditis.
- c i) Janeway lesions (non-tender; appear typically on the palms and soles).
  - ii) Splinter haemorrhages.
  - iii) Conjunctival haemorrhages.
  - iv) Roth's spots (fundal haemorrhages with central pallor).
  - v) Changing cardiac murmurs.
  - vi) Finger clubbing.
  - vii) Splenomegaly.
  - viii) Pallor.

The typical triad of infective endocarditis includes fever, 'embolic' phenomena and changing murmurs.

161 i) Reticulohistiocytosis.
- ii) Gout.

162 a Target lesions.
- b Erythema multiforme.
- c i) Herpes simplex.
  - ii) Mycoplasma pneumonia.

163 a Right oculomotor (third cranial nerve) palsy.
- b The pupillary fibres lying peripherally in the nerve are supplied by pial

blood vessels and so tend to be spared in ischaemic oculomotor palsies.

164 a Rheumatoid arthritis.
     b A shoe insole should be fitted. This should be modelled to provide support behind the metatarsal heads, thus taking weight off them.

165 and 166

     a i) Bilateral hilar lymphadenopathy.
        ii) Nodular infiltrates in both lung fields, predominantly in the lower zones.
     b Numerous punched out lytic defects; lacework reticulated pattern in the phalanges; some resorption of the distal phalanges.
     c Sarcoidosis.

167 and 168

     a Measles.
     b i) Koplik's spots.
        ii) They develop in the prodrome.
     c Lymphoid hyperplasia with multinucleate giant cells (Warthin-Finkeldey cells).

169 a A — Common bile duct.
        B — Gall stone.
        C — Portal vein.
        D — Inferior vena cava.
     b i) Endoscopic retrograde cholangiopancreatography.
        ii) Percutaneous transhepatic cholangiogram.
        iii) Intravenous cholangiogram. This is unlikely to demonstrate the biliary system unless jaundice is mild and/or resolving.

170 and 171

     a Vasculitis (causing ulceration, purpura).
     b These include
        i) Rheumatoid nodules.
        ii) Digital arteritic infarcts (usually around and under the nails, finger pulps: occasionally bullous, may become gangrenous).
        iii) Livedo reticularis.
        Neuropathic ulceration may occur secondary to vasculitic sensory neuropathy. Gravitational ulcers are more common in rheumatoid disease. Pyoderma gangrenosum has been described.

172 a Absent axillary hair.
     b Sheehan's syndrome (post-partum pituitary necrosis).
     c i) Failure of postpartum breast engorgement and lactation.
        ii) Failure of (shaved) pubic hair to regrow, failed growth/loss of axillary hair.
        iii) Continued amenorrhoea.
        (Other features of pituitary failure, eg hypothyroidism, if present at all, are usually late in onset).

173 a Scarring alopecia.
  b i) Secondary or tertiary syphilis (although the degree of alopecia seen here is rather extensive for secondary syphilis).
    ii) Systemic lupus erythematosus.
    iii) Leprosy.
  In ii) and iii), the VDRL test is falsely positive.

174 and 175
  a Granuloma annulare.
  b Diabetes mellitus.

176 a Atrial flutter with 2:1 block.
  b Beat to beat variation in intensity of the first heart sound occurs in atrial flutter.
  c Increase in the degree of AV block; and conversion to atrial fibrillation commonly occurs.

177 and 178
  a Perforating foot ulcer; gas in the soft tissues of the foot.
  b Diabetes mellitus resulting in a neuropathic ulcer with superinfection by gas-producing organisms.
  c Clostridium species or E. coli are the major causes of this appearance.

179 Degenerative disease of the lumbar spine. Ankylosing spondylitis may give rise to identical symptoms and signs, but is unlikely to present at this age.

180 a Loss of central vision with preservation of peripheral vision.
  b Congenital toxoplasmosis. Syphilis, toxocariasis or rubella are unlikely to cause such a well-defined, pigmented lesion.
  c No. Subsequent pregnancies are not affected.

181 and 182
  a Acute myeloblastic leukaemia, promyelocytic variant.
  b Disseminated intravascular coagulation.

183 a Subarachnoid haemorrhage with blood extending into the third and lateral ventricles.
  b Rupture of an aneurysm of the anterior communicating artery.

184 a The tympanic membrane is opaque and retracted, with a horizontal fluid level. Chronic secretory otitis media.
  b Bilaterally negative Rinne tests; Weber's test may lateralise if the severity of disease is unequal.
  c No. Autoinflation, Politzerisation, decongestants and myringotomy with or without grommet insertion are the basis of treatment.

185 a Bilateral ptosis, more marked on the left.
  b Myasthenia gravis.
  c Intravenous injection of edrophonium chloride.
  d No. Peak incidence in men is in the sixth and seventh decades.

186 a Pigmentation of the lips.
   b Gastrointestinal polyposis; Peutz-Jegher syndrome.
   c The risk of malignant change in the polyps is very low but such change has been recorded. In women, there is an increased incidence of ovarian carcinoma.

187 a Massive hilar, paratracheal and upper mediastinal lymphadenopathy.
   b Hodgkin's disease.
   c Nodular sclerosing (the most frequent variety overall).

188 a Knuckle (Garrod's) pads on the middle and ring fingers.
   b It may be inherited as an autosomal dominant condition or may arise spontaneously.
   c Dupuytren's contractures.

189 and 190
   a i) 'Calabar' swelling of left hand.
      ii) Soft tissue calcification.
   b Loiasis — caused by the filarial parasite loa loa.
   c Confined to Central Africa.

191 a Urticaria (with annular lesions).
   b i) Blood transfusion.
      ii) Dextran (40 or 70) transfusion.

192 a Iridodialysis.
   b i) Penetrating eye injury.
      ii) Surgery (eg. for glaucoma).

193 a Central cyanosis due to methaemoglobinaemia.
   b Sodium or potassium chlorate.
   c Intravenous methylene blue.

194 a Mumps meningitis.
   b Clear cerebrospinal fluid under normal pressure with a lymphocytosis, normal glucose and moderately elevated protein.
   c Paired serology to mumps S and V antigens.

INDEX

Acanthosis Nigricans 65
Achondroplasia 58
Addison's Disease 64, 153, 154
Adrenal Hyperplasia, Congenital 50
Alopecia 173
Alveolitis, Extrinsic Allergic 136
Amenorrhoea 22
Amyloidosis 6
Anaemia, Aplastic 15
Aneurysm, Ventricular 25, 79
Ankylosing Spondylitis 179
Arcus, Corneal 67
Argyll Robertson Pupil 13
Arteritis, Temporal 5
Arthritis, Gonococcal 52, 53
Arthritis, Rheumatoid 30, 69, 135, 164
Asbestos Exposure 98
Atrial Flutter 176
Beau's Line 118
Bleeding Disorders 29
Bronchiectasis 147, 148
Brushfield's Spots 41
Bursitis, Prepatellar 4, 93
'Calabar' Swelling 189, 190
Carcinoma, Basal Cell 36, 40
Carcinoma, Bronchus 73, 74
Carcinoma, Hepatocellular 56
Carcinoma, Squamous 111
Cataract 128
Cirrhosis, Primary Biliary 143
Coagulation, Disseminated Intravascular 181, 182
Coeliac Disease 57
Colitis, Ulcerative 157
Coloboma 100
Cranial Nerve Palsy, Accessory Nerve 146
Cranial Nerve Palsy, Oculomotor Nerve 163
Crohn's Disease 112
Cryoglobulinaemia 152
Dermatomyositis 109
Diabetes Mellitus 83, 128, 177, 178
Down's Syndrome 41
Dupuytren's Contracture 104
Dystrophy, Myotonic 62
Eczema, Atopic 46, 47
Edward's Syndrome 7, 8
Effusion, Pericardial 9
Ehlers-Danlos Syndrome 117
Emphysema, Surgical 68

Endocarditis, Infective 160
Epiloia 96, 97
Erythema Ab Igne 66, 99
Erythema Multiforme 162
Erythema Nodosum 112, 113
Erythema, Palmar 122
Factor VIII Inhibitor 29
Fracture, Scaphoid 89
Ganglion 95
Garrod's Pads 188
Gaucher's Disease 26, 27
Gingivostomatitis 55
Goitre 28
Glomus Jugulare 1
Gout 23, 24, 161, 60, 61
Granuloma Annulare 174, 175
Granuloma, Pyogenic 45
Graves' Disease 101, 144
Gynaecomastia 70
Haematoma, Intracerebral 92
Haemorrhage, Subarachnoid 183
Heart Block, Complete 71, 130
Herpes Simplex Infections 55, 11, 103
Herpes Zoster 146
Herpes Zoster Ophthalmicus 82, 108
Hodgkin's Disease 12, 187
Horner's Syndrome 19, 20, 116, 134
Housemaid's Knee 4, 93
Huntington's Chorea 54
Hyperuricaemia 23, 24
Hyperparathyroidism 126
Hyperviscosity Syndrome 16, 18
Hypoadrenalism 64, 153, 154
Hypothyroidism 77, 150, 151
Hypothyroidism, Juvenile 32
Ichthyosis 12
Iridodialysis 192
Keratoses, Solar 43
Knuckle Pads 188
Koilonychia 80
Koplik's Spots 167, 168
Kussmaul's Sign 51
Leishmaniasis, Visceral 2
Leukaemia, Acute Myeloblastic 181, 182
Leukaemia, Chronic Lymphocytic 86
Leukoplakia 72
Lichen Planus 105, 106
Loiasis 189, 190
Looser's Zones 42
Lymphadenitis, Tuberculous 145
Lymphadenopathy, Mediastinal 59

Lymphadenopathy, Hilar 59, 165, 166
Macular Degeneration 115
Marfan's Syndrome 120, 121
Measure 167, 168
Melanoma, Malignant 31
Meningitis, Mumps 194
Methaemoglobinaemia 193
Mountain Sickness, Acute 131
Muscle Dystrophy, Limb Girdle 34, 35
Myasthenia Gravis 185
Myxoedema, Pretibial 101
Naevus, Sebaceous 40
Naevus, Strawberry 10
Nelson's Syndrome 84, 85
Nephrotic Syndrome 159
Neuralgia, Post-Herpetic 123
Neurofibromatosis 90
Neuropathy, Ulnar Nerve 37
Nodes, Bouchard's 87
Nodes, Heberden's 87
Nodes, Osler's 160
Obstructive Airways Disease, Chronic
    138
Optic Atrophy 107
Osgood Sclatter's Disease 63
Osteoarthropathy, Hypertrophic
    Pulmonary 147, 148
Osteoarthrosis 87
Osteomalacia 42
Otitis Media, Chronic Secretory 184
Paget's Disease of Bone 119
Papilloedema 131
Pericarditis, Constrictive 51
Peutz-Jergher's Syndrome 186
Photosensitivity 38
Pityriasis Versicolor 102
Pleural Plaque 98
Polyartertitis Nodosa 75
Prader-Willi Syndrome 129
Pregnancy 22
Pressure Sores 6
Priapism 156

Proptosis 21
Pseudopapilloedema 14
Psoriasis 23, 24, 33, 139, 140, 141, 142
Purpura 81
Pyoderma Gangrnosum 157, 158
Renal Failure, Chronic 126
Reticulohistiocytosis 161
Rheumatic Fever 78
Rheumatoid Nodules 30
Ringworm 49, 91
'Rockerbottom' Foot 7, 8
Sabre Tibiae 119
Sarcoidosis 165, 166
Scrofula 145
Sheehan's Syndrome 172
Spinal Muscle Atrophy 94
Streptococcal Infection 78
Subacute Degeneration of Spinal Cord
    133
Swelling, Groin 137
Swelling, Neck 28
Syphilis, Congenital 119
Tamponade, Cardiac 9
Tendon Rupture, Supraspinatus 3
Thalassaemia, Major 39, 48
Thyroglossal Cyst 132
Tinea Cruris 91
Tinea Incognito 49
Toxoplasmosis 180
Trisomy 18 7, 8
Trisomy 21 41
Troisier's Sign 116
Tuberculosis 127, 145
Tuberous Sclerosis 96, 97
Turner's Syndrome 88
Ulcer, Neuropathic 117, 178
Ulcerative Colitis 158
Urticaria 191
Vasculitis 170, 171
Wernicke's Encephalopathy 149
Xanthomata 143